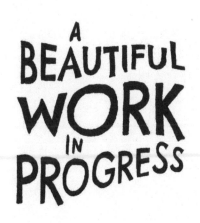

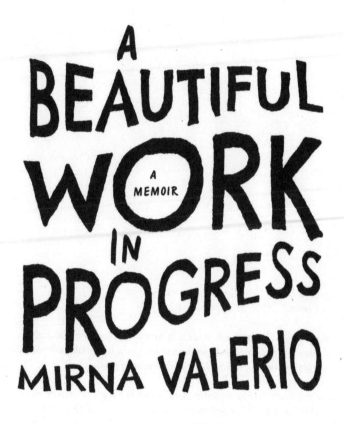

A BEAUTIFUL WORK IN PROGRESS

A MEMOIR

MIRNA VALERIO

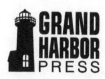

GRAND HARBOR PRESS

Published by Grand Harbor Press, Grand Haven, MI

www.brilliancepublishing.com

Amazon, the Amazon logo, and Grand Harbor Press are trademarks of Amazon.com, Inc., or its affiliates.

ISBN-13: 9781503943391
ISBN-10: 1503943399

Cover design by Faceout Studio

Printed in the United States of America

To my family, their legs, hearts, and spirits.

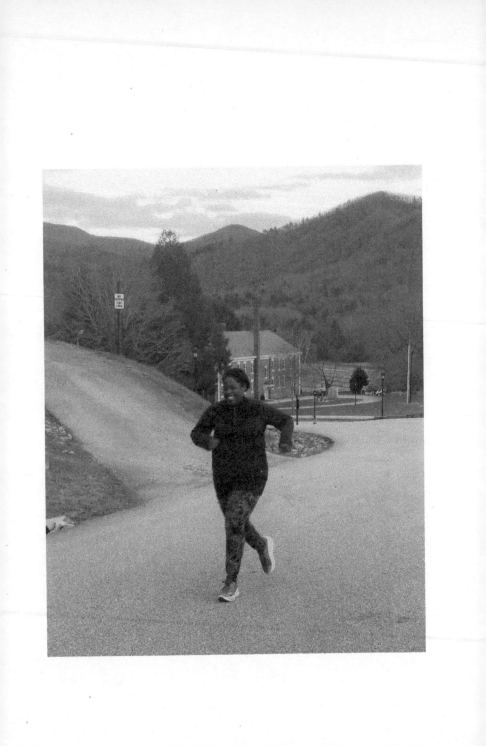

Teal, neon upper
Rubber chasing dirt and rocks
Soul on soul on sole

Kicking dirt, pebbles
Grooves in trails and mountaintops
Step over stepping

Searing desert hot
Arid cacti stinging hands
Stately saguaros

Prancing, jumping, go
Rock hopping, boulder stomping
A fat girl running

/

The Enablers

I sat on the king bed at the Best Western Mountain View in East Ellijay, Georgia, the night before the DoubleTap 50K race at Fort Mountain State Park in the Cohutta Mountains. It was late April and the entire month had been busy, what with rehearsals and preparations for my school's participation in the state's High School Musical Theatre Awards, two interminable days of tech rehearsals at the Cobb Centre in Atlanta, and an extremely long evening of awards, performances, and speeches. I had received a nomination for best musical director, but a veteran teacher won, deservedly so.

I was spent, extremely fatigued, and functioning purely on fumes. Okay, I wasn't that hopeful of completing the entirety of the next day's distance; nonetheless, I still had a race to at least *start* and experience.

My friend Kelly, whom I had met the previous year at the Nantahala Hilly Half Marathon in North Carolina, was with me. We'd struck up an immediate friendship at the back of the pack; we had to stick together. Who *else* can you commiserate with when you are at the tail end of a long stream of gazelle-like runners? At Nantahala, we cheered each other on, along with another friend-to-be, Ariel, and decided that we would call ourselves the Turtle Sisters.

As we sat on the bed, eating pizza (we had ordered a medium pizza to share, but somehow ended up with two extra-large supreme pizzas . . . you know, *carb loading*), we talked about our upcoming race plans, because that's what you do before the shock of finishing a difficult race wears off. She had recently registered for the Bryce Canyon 50M race in Utah, and I was deciding between signing up for another 50K or my first 50M.

After some serious, sleepy pondering, I decided that I wanted to celebrate the end of my thirties and the beginning of my forties in *style*. I wanted something different—out of the box and way out of my comfort zone. To many seasoned marathoners and ultrarunners, moving up on the distance continuum is a natural, logical step. You do a few marathons, and if you're a bit masochistic, you graduate to 50Ks and 50Ms, and then if you've really caught the ultra-bug, you take the leap to trying 100Ks and 100Ms. Some crazy folks go even farther, running a 135M race through the hottest days of the year in Death Valley (people such as Dean Karnazes of *Ultramarathon Man* fame; Cory Reese, blogger and author of *Nowhere Near First*; and Charlie Engle, the man who conceived of and executed a run across the Sahara) or running for 48, 72, or 166 hours at a multiday timed event.

The Javelina Jundred takes place in the outskirts of Phoenix, Arizona, over the Halloween weekend; the notion of running this race had been milling around in my head for the past few months, although I couldn't quite remember how it first entered my consciousness. Perhaps reading posts on the Trail and Ultra Running (TAUR) Facebook page and race reports had piqued my interest. Or it could have been someone's race T-shirt that had caught my attention. Somehow my curiosity was engaged, and I wondered aloud if I should go ahead and sign up for this crazy-sounding race, even though the distance was way beyond what I thought I could actually achieve. I had read about Jamil Coury, the owner of the race-management company Aravaipa Running, and the epic events that he had advertised in *Trail Runner Magazine* the previous year and was a bit afraid but expectant that I would be irretrievably sucked into the mysterious world of ultramarathoning outside of the East Coast.

"Should I do it? What if I can't? *Kelly! Tell me what to do!*"

"Do it," she said calmly, while completely absorbed in an episode of the popular 1990s-era sitcom *A Different World*.

I envisioned all the possible scenarios: training would be perfect and I would sail through sixty-two miles confidently albeit slowly; I would injure myself at a critical point in training and not be able to even start the race (in runner's jargon this is called DNS, or "did not start"); I would start training, lose motivation, and feel ashamed; I wouldn't start training because I couldn't wrap my brain around a distance larger than a 50K; or I would train, put in the work, have good days and bad days, get stressed out and overwhelmed with life and still have to train, and finally run the race.

In typical Mirna fashion, once I have weighed the pros and cons of a potentially life-changing decision, I open up to the universe or a friend and allow them to nudge me toward taking the proverbial plunge.

I took a deep breath and looked up at the ceiling, thinking *Should I? Shouldn't I?*

"Kelly, are you sure I should do this?"

"Yep. You already know what I think," she said in between bites of greasy, soggy, meat-heavy pizza.

"Okay, I did it." And then I gasped, realizing the magnitude of what I had just done. "Oh my God. I don't believe . . . Holy crap! What did I just do?" Inevitably, I asked myself this question after registering for most every marathon and ultradistance race.

Clicking the "Purchase" button on UltraSignup.com was too easy. There was even a button to share on Facebook what I had just registered for, and without much forethought, I clicked on that too. I added, "Shit just got real" to the prepopulated post that read "Mirna Valerio is now registered for the 2015 Javelina Jundred 100K. If you want to join, sign up now on UltraSignup." My ultrarunning friends understood the need to constantly push the envelope in pursuing the deepest end of your own personal running spectrum. Nonrunner friends asked if I was crazy.

Now I was committed—*all in*. Then the panic started to set in. *What had I just done?* I was suddenly full of questions that I probably should have asked myself before registering. *Will I be able to finish? Can I actually find time to train for this monster of a race? Will my big body be able to handle the requirements of the distance? Am I in over my head? Is this the event that'll prove how a fat person really shouldn't be running long distance?*

After I remembered that I had a race the next day, I closed my computer, finished my cold pizza, and got ready for bed. I tried to keep my mind on the enormous task that lay ahead at DoubleTap.

"You know anything about this course?" I asked Kelly, who had already tucked herself in. I hadn't bothered to look at the race website or read the race director's long e-mail.

"Something about a power line and nine thousand feet of elevation. That's what I read on the site. I hear it's kinda crazy."

"Great. Just great. Why do we do this to ourselves?"

With that, she snuggled into the cocoon she had made with the comforter and wished me good night.

The next morning we drove to the start line of the DoubleTap 50K at Fort Mountain in Chatsworth, Georgia. The rain loudly pelted Kelly's Nissan Cube, as it had on the drive up from Rabun Gap. We started the race after listening to the soft-spoken race director (RD) explain the slightly confusing course to us just one more time. The heavy rain continued as we made our way down the paved Forest Service road. We turned left into the forest and began the real adventure that awaited us.

I DNF'd, or "did not finish," in racing terms. I ran and hiked a total of twenty miles. The course was exceedingly difficult for me. I was slow from the beginning and didn't gain any momentum throughout the day. I was fatigued from the relentless pace of the previous weeks at school, and my legs and lungs would have none of it.

Meanwhile, Kelly finished with a great time for her first 50K. She beamed with a wide, satisfied grin as she made her way up the hill to the end, pumping her trekking poles all the way to the table where the volunteer would record her time and give her a finisher's pint glass. She was excited to have done so well on such a beast of a course, and was rightfully proud of her accomplishment.

"Hey—well done, Turtle Sister," I said as I embraced her tightly. She then sat down in a camp chair and drank some of the lukewarm pink electrolyte drink.

My experience at DoubleTap was vastly different. Both my body and mind had a tough time getting in gear. As for most of my races, there were sections of the trail where I sailed through (they weren't technical—meaning there were few rocks, branches, boulders, and other natural elements that hinder one's movement forward) and other sections, though technically difficult, where I managed to get through without pondering throwing myself off the nearest cliff. That said, something was still missing: the need and will to finish. I had nothing to prove to anyone. I knew that had I actually prepared for the race both mentally and physically, I might have had a different mind-set, but perhaps not. The following week at work would be full with more rehearsals, classes, arranging music for a beloved colleague's memorial service (a good bit of which I accomplished during my many hours alone on the trail), lesson planning, and meetings. The next morning I would take my choral group up the mountain to the next town and perform at a church service. I was already fatigued, and early on in the race I decided I would run and hike until I couldn't.

I met my first soul-crushing challenge thirteen miles into the hard-as-nails course. I had already done some cool rock scrambling on the scenic but highly technical Big Rock Nature Trail, hefting my legs over wet, slippery boulders (hence the name Big Rock), and at times having to do some low-level climbing on all fours to keep progressing forward. This part of the race didn't make me question my sanity. In fact, I enjoyed and looked forward to this kind of challenge, even with the stupor of lethargy that pervaded my entire being that day. From the trail I caught glimpses of the Cohutta Mountains through a filter of fog and stubborn stratus clouds, and the general dampness deepened the early-spring colors, their sharp vibrancy peeking out from under the cover of early afternoon mist.

A mile or two after leaving the Big Rock, a slight reprieve allows runners a few breaths before tackling the Power Line Climb. This infamous section of trail comes with its own cheery signage in all caps:

**POWER LINE CLIMB! WOO-HOO! BURN, BABY, BURN.
DT 100.**

This can't be a good sign, I thought. Someone had even decorated the two zeros of the "100" with googly eyes and a smiley face to laugh at us, someone who thought this was a good idea when we signed up and paid for this particular torture. Race directors of trail marathons and ultras tend to be sadomasochists, and many times are hell-bent on creating the most difficult courses to test both human body and spirit. This was one of them.

The Power Line Climb was exactly what its name suggested, a climb up a steep power cut. It began innocently enough, though. I thought, *This isn't too bad. It's a hill; I get it. That's what I signed up for.* But then the hill rose so sharply I imagined myself as a hunchback Sherpa carrying yak skins on my back. Yet I had just my hydration pack on, which felt like a filled-to-the-brim overnight backpack complete with sleeping bag and provisions. The climb was a mile long. It took me forty-three minutes to trudge slowly up the interminable hill.

The whole day the sky threatened to release a fury of thunder and lightning on us at any moment. Given that this part of the course was the slowest and most demanding, I resigned myself to death by electrocution should lightning strike one of the long wooden poles connected to each other by live wires. Electricity-filled lines whose continuous buzzing sounded like multiple swarms of angry bees surrounded me.

The only way to get up the mountainside was by moving slowly and deliberately. I hadn't thought to bring trekking poles with me. I hadn't ever needed them in a race. I would learn my lesson, however. When I finally reached the top of the climb, I was overjoyed and annoyed.

"Finally, goddammit. Shit! What the *fuck* was that?" I yelled to no one in particular, since I was alone, at the back of the pack. I hadn't seen anyone the entire time I traveled up the hill, and it was another fifteen minutes before I laid eyes on another human being. A race volunteer dressed in a bright-yellow T-shirt with the word "ENABLER" in big block letters across the front came running from the other direction. I quickly realized that he was coming for me.

"Hey, you okay?" he asked as he approached.

"I'm fine, but what the hell was *that*? That fucking sucked."

"Yeah, the Power Line Climb. At least you don't have to do it again." He chuckled.

"Well, even if I did, I wouldn't. That was really . . . what the hell was Perry thinking?" Before he could answer, I said, "I know, I know. I signed up for this. But damn."

He smiled again and extended his hand. "I'm Ric, by the way."

"Mirna," I said.

"I know. Lemme ask you a question. Where are your poles?"

"I didn't bring any. I mean, I've never used poles before, so it wasn't something I was thinking about. But I see my mistake. I've definitely learned my lesson. Never again."

"Here, try mine. They really help, especially on the long uphills like this. You use your entire body to propel you forward, so you're not as tired."

He handed me both poles and showed me how to loop the straps around my wrists. We then continued on the trail toward the next aid station, he without poles and me with poles, running up and down the rolling hills awkwardly at first and later with relative ease once I had settled into a rhythm—right foot, left pole, left foot, right pole. Using these advanced titanium versions of the hiker's walking stick helped with balance on tricky parts of the trail, and allowed me to spend more energy moving forward and less time worrying about whether I would face-plant onto the jagged face of a boulder. How had I never used these before? This was revelatory! My trail-running life would be significantly different from now on. I'd be a bit faster, and I wouldn't get fatigued so quickly. I felt I could tackle *any* race! Maybe not this one, though . . .

We chatted about ourselves. He was a local with a wife and children. He spent a lot of time out in these woods, running, volunteering, and doing trail maintenance. He pointed out the different types of trees and stopped before a tree with a large trunk.

"Do you know what that is?" he asked, pointing to the large opening at the bottom of the solid-looking trunk.

"Um, a hole?" I said, unsure of what he was getting at and embarrassed by my apparent lack of knowledge. Wasn't I already supposed to know these things? I mean, I spent a *lot* of time in the woods.

"That there is called a snag. It's when there's some kind of trauma to a young tree. But the amazing thing is that the tree keeps growing around the hole, despite what's happened to it. What's even more amazing is that the hole provides a home for animals and insects. Cool, right?"

"Wow!" I said, genuinely surprised.

"There are so many gifts in the forest."

We continued heading down the trail at an easy pace. I told him I was a teacher and that this race was supposed to be my third ultra, but I probably wouldn't finish. I didn't need the miles, and well, I was so tired I couldn't imagine trying to do the last ten-mile loop.

"Well, just do your best, and don't leave anything out on the trail," Ric said as we reached the point where we would go our separate ways. I returned his poles, and he bid me good luck.

"Bye, Ric! Thanks for helping me out and letting me use your poles!" But he was already gone, moving as quickly and efficiently as someone who *knew* their way around a trail.

The short time that I spent running with Ric renewed my faith in my body. Maybe, just maybe I could actually finish, even though deep down I knew the likelihood was pretty nonexistent. I continued on the course as it meandered its way through various trails in Fort Mountain State Park.

At about mile sixteen, the course went down a steep portion of the Pinhoti connector trail to a turnaround point where the runners were to choose a card from a deck on the side of the trail (I picked the jack of hearts). As I slowly made my way up the hill that seemed as though the trail gods had tacked on two extra miles just for shits and giggles, Ric came bounding down the trail again.

"Hey, you all right?" he asked, unsure if I was going to lie again about my well-being. "We were worried about you, and so I decided to see what was up."

"I'm okay. I'm just feeling real slow right now. Actually, I'm just not feeling it at all." He looked at me and silently handed me his poles. Who *was* this guy that kept saving me from myself?

We retraced my steps back uphill to the road that would bring me to the last four of the twenty or so miles that I would actually finish of the 50K course. At the top of the hill I ran into Crystal, another friend we had met at Nantahala, who had decided to call it quits at mile sixteen.

"Get it, Turtle Sister! You got this!" she yelled at the top of her lungs as she sat in the Swiftwick Socks car, recovering from the shock of those sixteen miles. I soldiered on, knowing that I had only a few more miles in my legs before I would call it quits. Ric's words echoed in my head, and I was determined to "not leave anything out on the trail." I ran for two more relatively easy miles until I hit the last aid station at mile eighteen, which was manned by two veteran trail runners, just on the verge of tipsy. At this point, there was a fork in the road: the trail on the left went uphill, and the one on the right was straight, flat, shaded, and inviting.

"Which way, friends?" I asked, munching on salty chips, Swedish Fish, and pickles.

"Well, if you want to get chased by a dog and shot at, go right. If you want to get to the next aid station, it's all uphill for the next two miles."

"You're kidding me, right? Like, seriously? What the . . . ?"

"Yeah, we know. But you're almost there," said one of them as he took a swig of some locally brewed IPA. "You got this, girl!"

I started up the trail on the left, which started switchbacking immediately, turning sharply to the left or right every tenth of a mile or so. I knew I wouldn't finish. One day I would complete the

DoubleTap 50K, but that day was yet to come. I focused all my energy on putting one foot in front of the other, stopping occasionally to adjust my pack, since my back and shoulders were becoming sore. I continued up the switchbacks, passing a low overhang, flat rocks jutting out from the hillside. I peered into the darkness below it and started walking faster. *Some unsavory person could be hiding in there.* I kept walking, swinging my arms in big arcs as though I had trekking poles. After I was a safe distance away from the dark space, I looked up and spotted a shadow ahead on one of the switchbacks.

Trail runners are known to mistake roots for snakes, low-hanging branches for aggressive buck antlers, and dark shadows for all manner of things. We become trail ninjas in the morning, swatting at spiderwebs with martial arts–like precision. We can also cower in the presence of large wildlife.

I thought I was hallucinating. *Did that shadow just move?* Nah, it didn't. I must be hallucinating. *Wait, did it just move again?*

"Holy shit, those are bears!" I screamed aloud. There were two adolescent cubs staring at me, curious. I stopped in my tracks and looked around. "Hello? Anybody? *Hello?* Is anyone here?" My heart was pounding. They seemed to be parked right on the trail, about a hundred feet away. "What should I do?" I asked myself out loud. I looked around and spotted a rock the size of my fist. I picked it up and grabbed the nearest stick I could find, my eyes on the bears the entire time. I blew the whistle attached to my pack and tooted a little ditty. Birds responded, but no humans did.

I started speaking to the bears, like any rational human being would.

"Hey guys, can you leave, please? Or can you at least, like, climb up into a tree so I can finish this damn thing? I just wanna go home! Seriously, bears, do me that favor, please."

They continued to watch me, and then both got on their hind legs and started whimpering, a sound much like a low-pitched whining from a dog. Then I started singing Rihanna at the top of my lungs. Still, they didn't move.

"Guys, come on! I just wanna go home, please? *Please leave!*" I yelled, waving my rock and stick frantically in the air.

Finally, I resigned myself to whatever fate lay ahead. I *had* to finish these last two miles and then get home to my boy. "That's all I want, guys! And I promise you I won't bother you anymore. Deal?" I started walking toward them, singing more Rihanna and waving my rock and stick. The trail traveled below them, and then it switch-backed above them. Their eyes followed me. Determined to lose sight of these ebony-colored fuzzy-wuzzies, I moved with a speed and agility that I didn't know I could have at mile nineteen of anything.

As I ran and power-hiked up the steep switchbacks, increasing the distance between the curious bears and me, I became uneasy again. *Did I just pass their den, and were those mom's eyes I had imagined peering at me from the depths of the dark below that rock overhang? She probably has her eyes on me right now. I'd better keep moving!*

As soon as I was far enough removed from bear danger, I breathed a sigh of relief. I wasn't maimed or dead. And it was actually kind of cool to have seen real live bears in their natural habitat. I also realized at this point that I was finished with my race. The bears had done me in. Any remaining energy stores I had were used up while freaking out about the innocent, curious bears. Even though I didn't have it in me to continue, I felt good about my decision. In less than a mile I would be done with the course, having left nothing out on the trail.

As I reflected on my race on the drive home, I agonized that I hadn't even wanted or cared to finish DoubleTap, what with its notorious Power Line Climb, all-around ridiculous vertical gains, and adolescent black bear cubs having playtime on the trail. I worried that giving myself permission to quit this race because it was too hard would set a dangerous precedent. I had just signed up for and relinquished my paycheck to a race that would be longer and certainly more difficult. Maybe I would give up in the middle of the Javelina Jundred 100K race and say, *Fuck it: I'm tired and I'm done.* Perhaps I had just wasted upward of $250 on the Javelina in a moment of utter stupidity. Maybe I would just take the loss, call it a day, and run my fifth Marine Corps Marathon on Halloween weekend like I had originally planned anyway. That would be easier.

Nope. I signed up for Javelina, and I wasn't about to waste my money. As I started strategizing about how I could finish a distance of this magnitude and not have the same outcome as I'd just had at DoubleTap, I embraced the excitement of this overwhelming challenge that I willingly subjected myself to and prepared to attack training with a fervor and energy I didn't know I could actually have at the end of an unbelievably stressful and anxiety-inducing school year.

———

Right after the Rabun Gap Nacoochee School let out in early June, I was free to begin a training regimen based loosely on Bryon Powell's book *Relentless Forward Progress*. I tried to keep my long runs on the weekends in tandem with his suggested length and frequency of back-to-back runs. I registered for several races, all of which would provide ample training mileage: the Tortoise and the Hare Ultra in Canton, Georgia; the Finger Lakes 50s 50K in Hector, New York; the Catamount 50K in Stowe, Vermont (I dropped down to the 25K—those *hills*); the Montour twelve-hour run in Danville, Pennsylvania; the Wildcat Ridge Romp 50K in Rockaway, New Jersey (I dropped down to the 10M option); and finally, the Georgia Jewel 35M run in Dalton, Georgia, at which I earned my second Georgia Jewel finisher's award, a heavy and giant engraved glass jewel.

Each race propelled me toward Javelina in different ways and taught me important lessons, the most important (well, I already knew this) being that Joann Taylor is the best mother, crew, and race-traveling buddy I could ever have.

From Tortoise and the Hare, I learned to run through the night without much stopping despite crushing fatigue, extreme humidity, and the onerous task of keeping myself entertained as I ran a flat one-and-a-half-mile loop multiple times.

At the Finger Lakes 50s 50K, a course that was composed of two undulating 16.5-mile loops, I discovered that I could keep going through calf-high mud, intermittent rain, general body grossness, mental fatigue, and a daunting second loop that was guaranteed to feel longer and be exponentially more difficult. Even though I checked my sanity at the beginning of the second loop, I knew I'd finish. Many folks decided to drop after the first loop, which was already a slippery and somewhat dangerous mud bath. The course would be even more treacherous, and it would prove nearly impossible to feel stable and grounded, particularly after hundreds of runners had already set foot on the compromised trails.

The Catamount 25K taught me that there is excellent trail running in Vermont. I wondered how I had *never* spent any significant time there, being a mountain-loving northerner and all. Even though those *verts monts* did a number on my legs, feet, and ankles, I gained a deep appreciation for Vermont's well-organized system of trails, many of which granted runners, hikers, and backpackers incredible vistas of rolling and craggy hills. I also learned that the Von Trapp family (as in the *Sound of Music*) is alive and well. They own the Trapp Family Lodge (where the race started) and have a successful brewery, which in the trail-running experience is an absolute must, particularly at the end of a grueling ultramarathon; a local IPA or summer ale is a tradition for many. Most importantly, the family, famous for its musical exploits, supports the trail-running, hiking, and cross-country-skiing community by sponsoring races and offering pristine and varied trails to adventure on. Perhaps most reassuring was realizing while in Stowe that trail folks are the same everywhere. Even if the aid-station fare (maple-syrup energy gels!) and trail talk change slightly by region, the pure and magnanimous heart of the trail-running community remains constant.

At the Montour event, my legs finally understood that they could still run at a fairly brisk clip after 26.5 miles on a 1.5-mile long loop without much pain or suffering. I also discovered that enjoying a wine festival at the same park that same day wasn't entirely bad—sangria and beer with lime at miles nineteen and twenty-three!

Wildcat, a difficult race put on by the owners of the New Jersey Trail Series and my good friends Rick and Jen McNulty, is always a crapshoot for me. I had run this particular event four times, and I never actually knew how many miles I'd eventually finish. The course is a 10M loop that features some difficult trail running and a slippery, mentally challenging stream crossing. I decided early on in the race that I would complete only one loop, have a beer, and then head home. I could have DNF'd early on at an aid station, but it helped to have Sal, the photographer from *NBC Nightly News*, trailing me that morning. At this race, I was reminded that it was impossible for me to beast through every race. This felt much like DoubleTap in that I had little will or need to finish. I learned to accept not finishing a particular event as a mode of self-care and injury prevention.

I hadn't planned on doing the Georgia Jewel, because I had *not* enjoyed running in the creepy forests of northwest Georgia for the ninety minutes it took to get through the all-uphill miles at the beginning of the course the previous year. Ric, my enabler from DoubleTap, suggested I try it again.

I knew that the Georgia Jewel (GJ) 2015 made the difference in my leg strength and physical endurance, along with massive improvements in perseverance and mental fortitude. The GJ is a challenging run on technical terrain, and I had sworn to myself after doing it the first time that I wouldn't try it a second time. After running, hiking, and slogging along for more than thirteen hours, I came in DFL ("dead fucking last," or in less shocking terms, "did finish last"). It had also taken me many days to recover mentally from having run alone in the dark for nearly two hours. After Ric convinced me to go for it a second time, I was more mentally prepared for the low points I would most surely have along the rolling hills of the Pinhoti Trail in northwest Georgia.

During one particularly bad moment, when I excoriated myself for letting Ric dupe me into climbing up and down slick mountainsides and rocky ridges, I stopped to gather my thoughts and steel myself for the next ascent. I looked down at my soggy trail shoes sinking in the mud and then up at the leaves that were just beginning their slow, yearly changeover to dormancy. I stood in the middle of the trail surrounded by occasional flashes of brick red, sunshine yellow, and burnt orange among damp dark-brown, almost-black tree trunks and tangles of bushes that existed in sharp contrast to the wet and pale-green tufts of grass that struggled to survive under the thick canopy of forest. I realized that I was fortunate. To be able to run freely and unencumbered on difficult trails in Appalachia was a gift.

"I am living the dream. I am *living* the dream!" I screamed to any tree that would listen. Here I was, huffing, puffing, and whining inwardly about something I had chosen to do of my own volition, about something I had the physical ability to complete. I made a silent promise to all my family members who had mobility issues, and to those who had heart disease and diabetes, that I wouldn't forget this. I was able. I was strong, and this little bit of suffering I could stand—for their sake.

I came up with several more mantras that day, born out of foot discomfort, chafing, long hours spent in my own head, and a sense of gratitude for each step, no matter the amount of pain. (I also discovered that postrace was an excellent opportunity to indulge in Panda Express Shanghai Angus Steak and copious amounts of greasy fried rice.)

I set out to tell anyone and everyone who would listen, including Clare Duffy, producer of *NBC Nightly News* (who had interviewed me that summer after *Runner's World* had done a feature on my running life), and various other media outlets that I was training for the Javelina Jundred 100K race. It became real. It became public. I would *have* to do it, unless I wanted to be the girl who said she would but then couldn't. I would have to prove to *myself* that this fat girl could keep moving for sixty-two miles, despite the internal doubt that pestered me from time to time, and despite the moments of fear that I would inevitably encounter both in training and during the event.

2

JAVELINA: HI, DESERT!

On the final day of October 2015, I stood at the starting line of Javelina, slightly chilled by the cold, dry desert air. I had stripped down to my thin tank (anticipating an intolerably hot day) and immediately started to shiver. Even though I knew intellectually that the desert is an icebox when the sun isn't up, the relatively cold air surprised me. I had harbored visions of a more Sahara-like experience, but it's probably freezing there in the mornings too.

I had no idea what to expect from running in the desert. Would I be running up and down soft and gently shifting sand dunes? Would there be scorpions and rattlers crawling about (I had been warned), or would my skin burn so much that I would look, as we used to say as young kids in Brooklyn, blue black or, even more descriptively, black and crispy? Did I have enough water, and would the aid stations run out before I got to them? Had I brought along the wrong electrolyte powder? *Was I going to die in the desert* and then never hear the end of it from my black friends and family as I lay in the grave?

All these questions milled around in my head as Jamil—the tall, curly-haired RD whose outward calm belied a fierce intensity and attention to detail—prepared to start the race. I don't typically get nervous or anxious at the start of a race because, hey, whatever happens happens, right? This time was different, however. I had basically announced to the world I would be *running* the Javelina Jundred 100K. So I *had* to do it, and I had to finish. In fact, there was no real question about finishing—barring injury, hypothermia, hyperthermia, or being burned to a crisp.

Numerous folks including family, real-life friends, social-media buddies, students, and colleagues had wished me well. They sent Facebook messages like "You got this, Mirna! Show 'em how it's done! One foot in front of the other! You've done the training, now it's time to enjoy the course! Do it with thy might!" I carried every one of them on my shoulders and in my heart that morning, and any self-doubt that had the nerve to show its ugly face was immediately crushed by this immense, positive vibe that I had been surrounded with in the months leading up to the race. I was going to make this happen no matter what.

Why am I doing this again? This is the question I always ask myself at the beginning of any distance event, which might be a 10M race or, in this case, a 62M race. Why am I subjecting myself to more than two consecutive marathons? Haven't I already done enough? And then I remember why I repeatedly throw myself into this pool of suffering—I love it. I love the experience of digging deep, pulling layer after layer off the onion that is me, discovering the most profound parts of myself over and over again.

While waiting for the inevitable, I took selfies and pics of the small crowd. I looked around and saw a woman whom I had "met" on Facebook.

"Are you Priscilla?" I asked a Latina woman clad in traditional trail-runner couture and accessories (hydration pack, capris, a technical tank top, and a Dirtbag Runners trucker cap).

"Hey! Nice to finally meet you," she said, hugging me.

"How're you feeling about this?" I asked, hoping she would be as nervous as I.

"Yeah . . . why are we doing this again?"

"I have the same question." We both chuckled knowingly.

A woman asked me to take a picture of her and her friend, and they did the same for me. Another runner caught my eye and told me that she followed me on Instagram and that she loved my feed. Could we take a selfie?

About two minutes before gun time (runnerspeak for the official start of the event), Jamil got our attention. Many of us fidgeted anxiously, tying and retying our shoes one more time, as we listened to his directions.

"Make sure you take care of yourself out there. Hydrate. Sunscreen. Rest when you need to. Visit the medical tent if necessary. Have fun. Run your own race. Enjoy our beautiful desert and mountains." After Jamil yelled "Go!" we set off. I was relieved to finally start but anxious for what the long journey ahead held for me. With sixty-two miles to go, I settled in with the rest of the back-of-packers until my body and mind were warm; I knew it would take me at least four miles to feel like I was in the zone, so I started slowly and deliberately, relishing the sensation of walking on a dusty terrain that was rather different than what I was accustomed to. The air was dry, and for this I was thankful I had brought two kinds of lip balm in the front shoulder pockets of my Nathan hydration pack. My nose, fingers, and earlobes were chilly to the touch, but I knew the air would warm and that the sun would eventually peek, then rise over the jagged peaks of the McDowell Mountains.

A little after the first two miles and after I had jogged some, testing out this sandy and gritty terrain, I stopped at the Coyote Camp aid station. The night before, after I had carefully and methodically set out my run kit for the race on the hotel bed, I reviewed the course map. Each loop was 15.3 miles long, and I would run four of them for the 100K distance. I knew to expect an aid station just a few miles into the run, but didn't fully understand its importance.

Wow, that's nice of them, I thought. *An aid station right at the beginning! Excellent choice of race, Mirna. This bodes well. This is going to be awesome!* I smiled a big smile and high-fived the nearest runner, a big guy also trying out his ultrarunning legs at the 100K distance.

"Yeah, man! Aid station. Woo-hoo! . . . Ooh: a Porta-Potty—gotta go!" Later on, this very aid station would be where I would begin my last, slow, pain-filled hurrah to the finish.

As I left the confines of the malodorous plastic privy (it had already been in use for the previous hour or so by the 100M runners), I joined a group that I had passed early on. One of them was Alicia, another runner who was similar in stature to me, though she was a bit shorter and thinner than I. She was on her second try at Javelina.

"Hi there!" I chirped, a little too perky for the early morning.

She responded with a little less enthusiasm than I thought was appropriate. "Hi."

"So how many ultras have you done? Are you a local? Have you done this course before?" My verbal diarrhea was astonishing even to me, but I figured if we were going to be in the back together, we might as well get acquainted.

"I made it two loops last year. I'm gonna try to finish this year," she said, keeping her eyes on the trail ahead. It almost seemed as though she wasn't interested in talking to me at all, but I kept at it anyway.

"Oh cool. Good luck! This is my first. I'm really looking forward to seeing how I do. I mean, I don't even know if I can finish, but I'm going to try to."

I have a tendency to gesticulate wildly and animatedly as I talk, even about banal things. I also lose track of where I am in space when I'm fully involved in an engaging conversation about something I love. Talking to people about running gives me energy, and my enthusiasm permeates my entire body.

"Shit! Ouch!" My left hand had brushed ever so gently against a pad of cholla cactus.

If you've never seen or heard of cholla cacti, let me take a few moments to explain to you how deceptively innocent they are. The desert is full of plants that live their long lives *daring* you to even look at them, threatening you with their long, spindle-like needles, and showing you who's boss when necessary. Animals have ways to simultaneously avoid and embrace these desert monoliths, and I would assume that locals in the area do the same to both evade and accept the majestic and mysterious saguaros and the cute, fuzzy, harmless-looking dwellers of the desert that jump onto and into you when you are least expecting it.

So much for innocent flora.

I hadn't realized that a cactus had actually attacked me until my nerves sent a message to my brain that dozens of inch-long needles had attached themselves to my index and middle fingers.

"Here, let me help you with that. There's a technique to this. It's gonna hurt a bit." Alicia, the taciturn local, picked up a small rock, careful not to brush her own body against any of the many cactus plants that surrounded us in every direction, and swiftly dislodged the cholla pad from my fingers in one fell, albeit painful, swoop.

I inhaled sharply and then recoiled again almost immediately when the cactus pad decided that instead of falling on the trail, it would veer left and attach itself to my foot, right through my fancy trail shoes.

Alicia was horrified. Now she was talking. "Oh my God, I'm sorry. I . . . I'm so . . . wow. Are you okay?"

I laughed it off (while wincing inwardly from the extreme discomfort of having several small stab wounds in my fingers). After I assured her that I was okay, I removed the cactus pad myself, the way she had done for my fingers.

"Thanks for helping me out. I would've hurt myself even more. Seriously, thanks. I appreciate it." I slowed down and allowed her some space to have her own experience.

I collected myself and continued on my way, speaking out loud to the desert. I didn't care who heard.

"Hi, desert! Thank you for allowing me to be here today in your beautiful expanse. I'm so honored to be in your presence, and I'm equally happy to have this opportunity to be here on your property. Thank you for hosting all of us, and I promise I will return the favor. But can you, like, not attack me with the cacti? I get it. I will honor you, and I know you are boss. But for real, though . . ."

By this point, I had started to warm up and get more accustomed to the fairly different terrain—dry and rocky with some damp spots. (I also didn't know the desert gets fairly frequent rain, but it dries up almost as quickly as it falls.) *This isn't so bad,* I thought. *I can handle this. No roots and branches to contend with, just fucking cacti.*

I had to make sure I didn't trip and fall over absolutely nothing, which I had a tendency to do, and ram into a saguaro (and get fined— since the late 1920s, it has been illegal to damage native plants on state-owned land in Arizona) or one of the other huge spindly plants that were only too happy to host a helpless human on their spindles.

Despite the cactus attack, the first loop was heavenly. The cool temperatures were perfect for this early-morning run. The heat wasn't oppressive yet, and I ran mostly unencumbered by roots and sudden dips and rises in elevation; the landscape was stunning; and the people at the back were pretty cool. We talked about our past accomplishments that year and our goals for the day (to finish, not to break an ankle like last year, to walk the entire distance in less than twenty-four hours), then wished each other well on our respective journeys.

As I finished the first loop, I was in high spirits. I felt strong and able, and I hadn't yet needed to use any of my mantras. I had taken my time at the aid stations, noshing on salty goodies, knowing that the day would be long and I needn't worry. I had set up my camp chair, gear, and food by the start line and was pleased to see that some anonymous soul had left a note with a cactus drawn on it, saying, "You're doing great!"

As I refilled my pack with energy gels and salty chips, Sarah, a woman whom I had met earlier in the day as I was setting up, came over to check on me.

"How's it going?"

"So far so good. I actually feel great. Like, the first loop almost felt easy." I beamed.

"Do you have a crew?" she asked.

"Nah. I didn't really want to ask anyone to come and hang out in the desert for an entire day with nothing to do."

"Well, I can crew for you! My sister's out doing the 100-miler, and I'm happy to crew for you while I'm still here. How about it?"

I was stunned by her generosity. "Really? I mean, that would be great, but if it's an imposition . . . that's really nice of you. Seriously."

"I meant what I said. What do you need now?"

"Wow. I really appr—"

"It's not a problem at all. I'm already out here, and you're here alone. And did you say this was your first time in Arizona? Happy to do it. So what do you need? A sandwich? Coke? Fruit? Gels?"

"Some Coke would be great," I said, still taken aback by her simple act of kindness. Sarah jogged over to Jeadquarters and returned with some flat Coke, a gel for "just in case," and a couple of gummy bears.

After I assured her that I was okay, I thanked her profusely, did a brief mental and physical assessment, and headed off to start my second loop. *Did I feel good?* Yes? *Could I do another loop no problem?* Absolutely. *Did I still enjoy running?* Yes. *Was I sufficiently hydrated?* I think. *Any pain in the body—knees, hips, feet, brain?* Not yet. *Still happy?* Yes.

I set off on my second loop and took out my phone to catch the stunning beauty of the trail, the sun, and the relief of having some mileage behind me. Forty-five miles left to go, and I still felt golden. I leapfrogged with my new trail friends, twins from Minnesota with thick midwestern accents who would carry identical gray parasols throughout the entirety of the three loops they would complete, for the next eight hours. Some other folks who had started in the back with me dropped out after the first and second loops. Devon Yanko, the tall and exquisitely run-chiseled woman who would win the 100M race in fourteen hours and fifty-two minutes, would lap me several times throughout the day (and evening), politely saying, "On your left" or "Excuse me" each time. I have this habit of following in people's footsteps for twenty or so run-steps at their same cadence, just to see how far I can get at their pace (not too far). I did this every time she passed me, sometimes twice during one loop, except for during the last few miles of my third loop.

Although the second loop wasn't easy per se, it hadn't been impossible either. There had been some challenges—mainly boredom and the occasional wave of dread about the distance before me, but I was still filled with energy and enthusiasm. Even though the sun had risen over the mountains and its rays beat down on us with an intensity only a desert sun could have, I welcomed the heat with an open heart. I'd signed up for this, so I wasn't going to complain about it. I imagined the sun ridding my brain of any negative thoughts I might have about the next thirty-one miles. I would be running in the complete darkness of a desert with whom I had just become acquainted. I would have to engage the third loop with survival tactics that I had planned well in advance to get through what would prove to be the most mentally painful part of the day. Loaded onto my phone were a few audiobooks: Travis Macy's *The Ultra Mindset*, Brené Brown's *Rising Strong*, and Chrissie Wellington's *A Life without Limits*. Playlists on my son's iPod included Drake, Indigo Girls, Missy Elliott, T-Pain, Simon and Garfunkel, Blind Pilot, Manu Chao, and the Cranberries. I planned to employ every tactic I had to get through whatever extreme lows and periods of self-doubt I would experience.

Before I set out for the third loop, I peeled off my dusty socks and switched them for a fresh pair, changed my shoes to the looser and less minimalist Pearl Izumi Trail M2s, slapped on some more of my magical lube concoction (Vaseline, Squirrel's Nut Butter, and Body Glide all mixed together), and sat down to rest and collect myself for a few minutes.

Adrian, an event manager for Altra Running, one of the race's sponsors, walked over to me. He'd also figured out that I was sans crew.

"Do you need anything?" he asked. I had noticed him watching me from his post with increasing curiosity as I came in from my first and second loops.

"No, I think I'm good," I said. "But thanks so much."

He ignored my response and went off to get some pizza, fruit, and flat Coke for me. The temperature would be dropping soon, and he knew that I would need the calories for warmth and sustenance.

When he returned, we talked about shoes and gear, which races I had done, and which ones I was planning to do in the future.

"So what are you wearing?" he asked, making a show of eyeing my shoes. I still had on my Pearl Izumi sneakers.

"Ha-ha! Don't worry. I've got my new Altra Olympus for the last loop. I got a plan, bro."

"I don't even have those. They're not even out yet!" he said, faking jealousy.

"I got mad connections," I said, jokingly.

"Well, let me know if you need any shoes or anything today. I'm happy to get you whatever you need."

Adrian is a sweet and kind soul, whose sheer generosity uplifted me and helped to set a strong mental tone for what would prove to be the most difficult part of the course for me. I went into purgatory with a sense of gratitude (and dread, I'm not going to lie), a renewed spirit, and a full belly.

The third loop was just as I had anticipated. Even though many people were still running in both directions (i.e., washing-machine style, wherein each loop was run in the opposite direction), I felt as though I were out there alone. Staying focused on the task became more and more difficult. As the miles went by, I became lonelier. At times, the only other living beings around were the imposing saguaro cacti and an occasional spindly animal scurrying across the trail. Some runners stopped to take long naps (I almost tripped over a guy snoozing at the side of the trail), thus distorting our leapfrog game. Other runners stopped, entirely satisfied with their mileage, whereas others were exhausted beyond belief, DNFing just as the statistics from previous years said they would.

I ran and walked alone for long stretches of time through the night until someone came running from the opposite direction. *This must be what it's like to be on the moon,* I thought. Seeing other humans became increasingly important to me during the wee hours of the morning because the dark desert night felt progressively desolate and foreboding. Until the moon showed her face, I felt like I had entered an airy mine in which headlamp-clad workers would periodically come at me from ahead and behind, startling me out of my own head.

Two hours into the third loop, I discovered that my fancy wave-on, wave-off lamp had actually been turned on while it had been in my bag at the starting line, causing the battery to die during the darkest part of the evening (post-sundown, pre-moon). I was stranded. I suddenly lost all sense of direction and spatial reasoning. There were no other runners around, no sounds, no tiny beams from faraway headlamps. I sighed. *What to do?* The only option short of making potentially dangerous navigational mistakes and crashing into more cacti was to wait until other 100K and 100M runners on their fourth, fifth, and sixth loops passed me from behind. I would then be able to follow them and their half-moon auras for a few minutes until I couldn't keep up anymore. At least I would be moving forward, continuing the journey—albeit much more slowly than I was already traveling. This plan would bring me closer to Jackass Junction, the midpoint aid station where most of us had stored necessary provisions and where I could retrieve the extra headlamp I had stowed in my drop bag.

At one point, I stopped dead in my tracks. No one seemed to be coming or going. I took a deep breath and resolved to keep moving forward, even with the risk of a second and third cholla-cactus attack. I didn't care. I *had* to get to Jackass. Just then, a runner who moved toward me from the opposite direction was startled by my presence in the desert darkness.

"You all right?" he asked.

"Well . . . no."

"What's up?"

"My headlamp burned out," I said, frustrated with myself for having apparently overlooked the possibility of having a nonfunctioning headlamp.

"That's a bummer! Do you have an extra?"

"Yeah, I do, but it's at Jackass."

"Listen, I have an extra flashlight that you're welcome to use."

"Oh my God, really?" Having long, drawn-out conversations in the middle of the night wasn't exactly easy after having been moving for more than eighteen hours.

"Yeah, just leave it in my drop bag at the start when you're done. No worries."

"Oh my God. You're so sweet. Your name?"

"Ray."

Like Ray's Pizza in New York. Ray Charles. Ray Liotta.

"Thanks so much, Ray. Like, really. Thank you so much!"

Trail magic happens most unexpectedly and when most needed. Ray had given me a lifeline and a much-needed boost of mental energy. I now could continue to the aid station (albeit slowly and with some hallucinating), replenish my energy stores (food, good feelings, gear, lube), and then keep moving forward. I was five and a half miles away from the next station, and so far those miles had been the most difficult of the night. Even though I had left the first aid station feeling fairly awesome, I quickly realized that I still had many, many more miles to go.

I would have to run, walk, crawl, death-slog, and slowly inch my way forward through the night, ignoring my already out-of-sync circadian rhythms and precious sleep cycles, into this unknown territory that I would become quite familiar with through the nearly twenty-six hours it would take for me to reach the finish line. I would have to finish traversing this 15.3-mile loop, and then do it again. Although the loop had been an uplifting and hopeful new beginning in the brilliant morning and afternoon light, it would be downright shudder-inducing in the fully enveloping and stunningly claustrophobic darkness of the desert night. The headlamp incident paled in comparison to what was next.

A herd of growling javelinas was coming to get me. The javelinas' menacing oink-grunts grew louder and more intense as I rounded bends on the course and climbed dusty, pebbly hills among light-absorbing, looming saguaro and vicious cholla cacti.

"Did you guys hear that?" I asked a struggling runner and her pacer, the woman whose job it was to keep her runner on course, at a strong pace, and sane.

"Hear what?"

"The animals? The ones, um . . . growling?" I said, realizing I might sound crazy.

"Um, no?" They continued on, the thin, fresh-legged runner reminding her charge that she *had* to eat something before the next aid station, which seemed like it was an eternity away. They ran off, the overly perky pacer a few steps ahead of her delirious runner.

I definitely heard growling, I thought. *I am* not *crazy.* What else could that noise be? I couldn't have been the only person who could hear the fairly consistent, low-pitched slow rumble that sounded as if these piglike animals were planning their attack, timing their oink-growls to each of my Pearl Izumi–clad steps.

This must be why this race is called the Javelina Jundred! It was an epiphanic moment. What makes this race so *special* is that runners get to hear and possibly encounter actual javelinas. *Wow!*

The low rumble continued in an almost conversational way. The sound would start as a barely audible but insistent hum and grow in intensity until the whole lot of javelinas had agreed on their plan to ambush the runners that night and leave their stinking, lifeless bodies to dry and disintegrate in the arid desert heat. I envisioned wild boars with large, yellow nutria-like teeth darting about, not much unlike Templeton the rat from *Charlotte's Web*.

Wait a minute! Why isn't anyone talking about or cowering in fear from these wild animals? Can't everyone hear them? Everyone else on the course must be a veteran of the race. No one had ever mentioned this in any of the prerace communications. *Can't wait to write my race report.*

I imagined coming upon human skeletons and screaming, gasping, and fainting in horror after the sun started to rise. Fortunately, both common sense and reason interrupted my auditory hallucinations. Let's see, on my first *two* loops, I hadn't seen any human skeletons in the daylight. Second, no one else seemed to be bothered by the so-called growling, menacing as it was. Third, not even *one* javelina jumped out from behind a saguaro to attack me. Fourth, the chorus of growling javelinas had a rhythmic quality to it.

It wasn't until many miles later, when I rounded a bend in the trail near the Rattlesnake Ranch aid station, the last one before reaching Jeadquarters, that I learned what was causing the noise: headlights and taillights from a few cars that had been on the desert roads for the previous few hours doing who knows what, drifting, speeding up, slowing down . . . doing what people do in cars in the desert in the middle of the night enveloped by dark sky.

But miles before this discovery, as I approached Jackass Junction, I heard pulsating, bass-heavy music coming from what sounded like a rave, a music-and-dance oasis in the middle of the desert. People sang and laughed loudly. I kept trudging on, closer and closer until I could see the light emanating from the many lines of twinkling bulbs that hung around the medical tent and a small enclosed area that resembled an outdoor-wedding dance floor.

The aid station appeared like a mirage in an old Bugs Bunny cartoon. I crested a small hill, and there it suddenly appeared. I thanked the universe and quickened my step; I couldn't get there fast enough. After collecting my drop bag from the neatly arranged bags just a few feet from the aid station, I plopped my heavy self onto one of the cheap plastic folding chairs across from the tables stocked with a variety of trail goodies that had changed according to the temperature. There was hot broth, ramen, tea, and coffee available to help runners maintain body heat during the night. A few runners rested under heavy blankets in the medical tent, warming themselves before attempting the next few miles.

I put my feet up on another chair, leaned back, and breathed deeply, inhaling the scent of wood smoke coming from the nearby fire pit. The tip of my nose was chilly, and I shivered a bit. Even though I had no intention of putting any food item near my lips, I knew that I would need to ingest some calories to stay warm through the cold, cloudless night. My stomach had shut down during the first few miles of the third loop, through the headlamp debacle, refusing most food and allowing only a painfully small amount of hydration in.

Jake, one of the volunteers, a dark-haired, bearded guy who fit the stereotype of trail runner—he wore old trail shoes held together by duct tape, a long-sleeved technical shirt from some trail race out west, and hiking pants—came over to me and asked what I needed.

"Ugh, I can't even stomach anything right now, and I'm totally bonking," I said.

"I know exactly what you need. Hold on. I got you." He jogged over to the table and filled up two cups, one with salty chicken broth and the other with ramen noodles in broth. "Drink the plain broth first," he said, standing over me to make sure I actually drank the nasty hot water.

"This is gross. But I know, I know!" I said, swallowing as quickly as I could so I wouldn't smell or taste the artificial chicken flavor.

"Now eat this." He took the first cup from my hands and replaced it with the second. Again, he made sure I slurped every last bit of the thin, curly noodles before walking away to refill my bladder with electrolyte fluid. Jake returned with my pack and some ginger slices covered in crunchy sugar.

My mind cleared suddenly and my stomach unknotted itself just as quickly. I sat up, feeling like a mortal morphing into her superhero. The contrast of black sky and twinkling lights was so sharp, I squinted my eyes. My feet stopped hurting, and when I stood up, I no longer felt woozy and disoriented.

"Hey, are you ready to go? You should get going. The longer you stay here . . ."

"Yep! I seriously feel like a new person. Thanks for being out here! 'K, bye!"

Before heading out, I crunched on some of my own jalapeño chips and stuffed two gels into my hydration vest pocket. I was ready to go, prepared to conquer the next six or so miles until the next aid station.

I referred to this part of the course as "Stover," as in the Stover Creek portion of the Pinhoti Trail. Stover is the part of the Georgia Jewel course that is seven long, never-ending, rolling miles of solitude and in-your-head-ness. In the grand scheme of things seven miles isn't a great distance to traverse, but in the moment (or after many hours) it feels as though you're trudging your way through the entirety of the Sahara with the world on your shoulders.

I made my way back to Jeadquarters with a smile and some relative pep in my step. Only one loop separated me from my epic personal finish.

3

The Wall Looming before Me

"Okay, who's next?" the guide asked, looking around at the few of us who were left standing at the bottom of the rock-climbing wall. I raised my hand timidly.

"What's your name?" asked the hiking pants–clad guide. He had a ring of carabiners attached to his harness, with various loops hanging from his hip belt.

"Mirna," I said nervously.

"Okay, Mirna, it's your turn. You ready?"

"Sure," I replied nervously, looking around at all my peers who had already climbed up the wall and rappelled down successfully. I could do this. It didn't look easy, but I could do it.

I lifted my right foot to the nearest hold, stretched out my right hand to a hold above my head, and began to lift myself up, very slowly. After about three seconds, my hands gave out, shaking, because I had hung the weight of my entire body on my hands and had no clue what to do with my feet. I dropped to the ground. "Climbing" and "On belay!" Same thing. There was silence from the guides and the rest of the students who were waiting below. I made it to one more dirty yellow hold, and then I promptly lost touch again.

In the final weeks of summer in 1989, there I stood in front of a rock wall in the middle of the woods somewhere in Connecticut, with fifty-nine other students from New York City, ready to embark on my first year at boarding school. Some of the students would travel to New England to settle into such storied campuses as Phillips Exeter Academy, Choate Rosemary Hall, and Miss Porter's School. Others would head to the mid-Atlantic to attend St. Andrew's, whose campus was the set for my favorite film, *Dead Poets Society*. I'd be attending the Masters School, a small all-girls school not far from New York City.

Our close-knit group was undertaking our final, formal bonding opportunity with icebreakers, low ropes, high ropes, and fear-inducing, physical strength–testing courses to help us function more effectively as both individuals and as a group. The retreat's purpose was also symbolic. The message was simple: we could do anything we set our minds to, no matter how difficult and overwhelming. Maybe we wouldn't be able to do it on the first try, but we'd better at least try our damnedest.

After we had completed the requisite tasks for both high and low ropes, our final challenge loomed in front of us down an offshoot trail: a huge wooden structure that had various colored and differently shaped objects screwed into it. We were supposed to climb this wall, using the shapes (holds, I later discovered)—the yellow ones if we felt we needed an easy route, and the red or blue ones if we were feeling strong. The guides, two scruffy white dudes in synthetic hiking pants who would be our leaders the entire weekend, harnessed us into straps and ropes. We practiced yelling "Belay on!" "Climbing!" and "More slack, please!" We learned that being the belay person didn't mean that you were responsible for all the weight of the person climbing, which was a relief for me, knowing that I was the heaviest person in the group and that belaying for me wouldn't really pose a hazard to anyone else or prevent me from at least trying.

The wall that stood before me was inviting but also invoked in me a new kind of fear. The sense of fright wasn't so much from the thought of hanging from the top of a very tall wall—I was okay with that—but the possibility that I wouldn't be able to haul my big ass up the wall that was looming before me. I feared I would fail. Even though we had been hiking fairly easily (and quickly) up and down hills, across streams and rickety bridges, this would pose a new challenge. I had already had some trouble hoisting myself over big boulders that my classmates had effortlessly pulled themselves up on earlier that day on the trail. Two boys, Jay and Cory, jumped back down from atop a boulder smack in the middle of the trail to help push me up. I held on helplessly to the guide's hands at the top and felt ashamed.

"On belay . . . ?" I said too quietly. No one heard me. I took a deep breath, paused when my lungs were full, and then yelled, "On belay?!" looking back at the group of my peers.

"Belay on!" the guide and students who were supporting me with ropes responded.

"Climbing!" I continued.

The belayers responded with "Climb away!"

I reached for the first yellow hold and immediately succumbed to gravity and a complete lack of upper-body strength.

I simultaneously hated and revered ropes courses. It always became clear rather quickly who was deemed a leader, who the docile herd of sheep, and who the dead weight. I always felt like a dead weight because I was not only heavy but also simply uninterested in taking on the kinds of leadership roles that were deemed the most valuable. I also didn't have age-appropriate social skills. I was *great* with adults, though. I wasn't witty, and I often was very blunt, not yet having refined my sense of tact, and this was definitely not helpful in most adolescent social situations.

"Okay, Mirna, let's try it again," the guide said encouragingly. I wasn't embarrassed yet. Other students had tried once and failed, so there was a precedent. I wasn't worried about that first try.

"On belay!"

"Belay on!" the group yelled cheerfully.

"Climbing!" I said, confidently this time.

"Climb away!"

This time I was able to grab on to the first yellow hold, then a green one. I lifted my left leg, but my hip cramped up just as I tried to push off.

"Ugh! Shit!" I said, disappointed in myself.

"Don't worry, Lady Guinevere! You can do it!" I chuckled and smiled. Tamia, one of the smartest and most vocal leaders of our cohort, had given us all names from the Knights of the Round Table. Even though Guinevere wasn't the greatest character with the most positive story (she'd had an affair with Sir Lancelot), I enjoyed being part of this social group, despite the artificiality (and nerdiness) of it all.

We went through a third series of climbing call-and-response, and I looked up at the wall, which seemed slightly less imposing now that I was Lady Guinevere, and tried again. This time I was able to reach one more hold, but my hands started shaking violently and I promptly lost touch with the hold and fell down.

Now I was frustrated and embarrassed. Lady Guinevere, the temptress and opportunist (I was neither), couldn't do it. But I was determined to try one more time. And I would come up with a plan before trying again.

I was usually slow to come up with a solution, preferring to process in my mind rather than talk it out. I conceptualized problems and solutions without communicating them out loud until I was finished solving a problem. I deliberated until a fully formed idea reared its head in my brain, complete with detailed compartmentalization, outlines, and flowcharts. And I needed to do it in silence, with zero pressure and no watchful eyes. Not an especially helpful technique in these situations.

But, of course, the reins were handed to the dominant loud talkers who needed to verbalize their ideas first. They were quick and efficient with their decision making, and I was not. These "team-building" activities only reinforced this. I was tired of relearning *who* was a leader and who was *not*. We all knew who they were, so why bother? We deferred naturally to those kids anyway.

These activities weren't a complete loss, however. I learned more about myself and what I was actually good at, even though the other half was learning over and over again what I was terrible at. I loved helping lift people through the spaces in the web of strings without touching the sides on the low-ropes course. I could do that. I loved encouraging my peers who were afraid of heights and hesitated on the ladder up to the zip line. I delighted in not having any fear of heights when others did. I felt an exhilarating release jumping off the platform (while harnessed, of course) to fly across the lake on the zip line, carabiner and cable zipping rhythmically as I traveled over the water, the humid air hitting my face, making my skin cool. I wasn't afraid. In fact, I craved being able to show people who didn't really know me that I was good at this. That although I wasn't useful socially, I was good at something besides math, science, and awkwardness. I excelled at jumping or hanging and zipping along a cable with the knowledge that I was tethered to only a thin rope with a deep lake below. I wasn't afeard of jumping off the Tarzan swing, or of traversing narrow rope bridges hung between small platforms way up in the trees. During those challenges I felt invincible and powerful.

I discovered my strength and my own personal brand of leadership in my outwardly carefree (but inwardly calculating) attitude toward things that to many seemed risky or dangerous. I was quiet and never felt a compelling need to be a leader in the bombastic and bossy way that many of my peers were.

For the fourth and final attempt at climbing that wall, I took half a minute to figure out my plan.

The wall stood there, imposing. I wanted to succeed so badly. I wanted to show everyone that I could do this even if I needed a little help and a few more tries. Academic subjects came easily. I could do advanced math, albeit quietly and slowly. I excelled at it. I could read medical tomes for hours on end without as much as looking up from the book or taking a break to use the bathroom. I could write a great essay on adolescent sexuality, do a fantastic history presentation on Plato's "Allegory of the Cave" with appropriate visuals . . . but I was losing faith that I could do this seemingly simple task.

Now I was frustrated. Couldn't the guides talk me through this, show me what I was doing wrong? I obviously needed help. It had looked doable from afar, from watching how everyone else had struggled a bit in the beginning but were eventually able to reach the top. I felt as though my body had failed me. I could run up and down the block all day, swim in a lake for hours, ride my bike around Bushwick, Brooklyn, from morning until evening, but I couldn't do this.

I stared at the wall in front of me. I looked it up and down, eyeing all the "easy" yellow holds. I had a plan. I would step up with my right foot first so I could be better balanced and not have all my weight on one side. I was going to do this. I took a deep breath and approached.

Before I could execute my plan, the guides warned me that other people were waiting. I could have one last try, and if I didn't succeed this time, I could just climb the ladder on one side of the wall, and rappel off the top on the other side. Any lingering determination I had as I looked up at the top began to dissipate.

Deflated, I decided I would only try to make it as far as that stupid yellow hold. *"Climbing!"* (I should have yelled *"Failing!"*) *"On belay!"* everyone said cheerily and, did I detect, wearily? I fell again, this time rushing to remove the carabiners and ropes from my hip belt. I walked around to the ladder without a sound, eyes watering, hooked back in to another set of ropes, and climbed up. My arms shook badly, but I managed to hoist myself up this ladder. A double failure would be crushing.

"This is the fun part," the guide stationed at the top of the wall said, smiling gently. "Just hook in, lean back, and use your feet to bounce down the wall."

"Okay. I think it got it," I said, and I did. I felt calm and capable. At least I could do this.

4

Do It with Thy Might

My mother watched us from the picture window of the Cameron Mann Dining Hall on the nonforested side of the too-short field-hockey field. All of us new girls had arrived that morning to begin our tenures at the Masters School, and we were out on the field waiting for the next instruction in our icebreaker activities.

Most of the other parents had left campus in their own cars. Some still lingered on the edges of the field, but eventually managed to tear themselves away from their daughters at this new juncture in their lives. Although the window had a glare, I knew it was her. I could see the outline of her hips as they abutted against the thin bright-purple cotton of the matronly shirtdress she had worn to bring me to school. I felt her watching me with pride as I got to know the other girls on the field.

I worried about her finding a ride to the Dobbs Ferry Metro-North train station. She assured me that she would be fine and that I shouldn't worry about her, but I did. This was it. I would no longer be living at home. I'd be ensconced in the rolling hills of Westchester County, part of the privileged few who got to attend boarding school. I wondered how she would get there—I was so distracted by worrying that I missed the instructions for the next activity because I kept looking up at the dining-hall window. She waved me off every time I raised my head to see if she was still there.

"Hey, Mirna, you okay?" asked one of the teachers leading our group.

"I don't know how my mother's going to get back to the train station," I said, looking up at her one more time. She waved at me again, and I knew instinctively that she was telling me to pay attention.

"Oh, I'll see if I can get someone to give her a ride," said the woman who I would learn was one of my dorm parents, Ms. O'Leary.

We didn't know anyone yet because I was a brand-new student at the school, and I knew my mother was too shy to ask for help. She always found a way to get things done on her own, but I felt like I had left her alone in a sea of wealthy, mostly white people.

We had taken a cab earlier that morning, with a surly, cigarette-smelling driver in an old '80s Ford, up the hill to the school for registration. We carried an assortment of big and small bags, anything that could hold stuff that we had found lying around our apartment, and packed the mound of stuff tightly onto a luggage carrier, held in place by a few colorful bungee cords.

After the cab had deposited us in front of the main building, the facade of which was weathered stone and brick, we followed the registration signs to the Claudia Boettcher Theater and opened the heavy glass doors, struggling to get our ragtag selection of bags and bungees through.

"Welcome to Dobbs!" said the thin, dark-haired woman who had interviewed me months before. Ms. Atlee was a young admissions officer at the school and seemed delighted to see me. She hugged me and shook my mother's hand.

"We're so glad you're here, Mirna! This way . . ." She motioned for us to follow her to the tables lining the long beige hallway outside of the theater.

Ms. Atlee called over a girl dressed in a white "Dobbs Gold Key" T-shirt.

"Hey, can you help Mirna and her mom with registration?" Ms. Atlee asked.

"Sure!" chirped the perky girl. *Everyone here is so perky and energetic,* I thought. She extended her hand and introduced herself. "I'm Amy. I'm a sophomore, but this is my third year here. And yeah, we're happy you're here. Did you have a long trip?"

"We came from Brooklyn on the train," I said, proud.

"Oh wow, you carried all of your stuff on the train?" she asked, incredulous.

"Yeah. We don't have a car . . . well, um, also, nobody in the family drives."

"I'm impressed. Let's get you all registered and everything, and then you can go see your room."

We went from table to table, introducing ourselves several times to an assortment of people. A tall older woman in a flowery flowing dress came over after she heard another woman say my name as she was flipping through the files to find my schedule.

"Hello! Mirna?" She extended her hand to my mother. "I'm your adviser, Mrs. Edmonds. So nice to finally meet you. We're excited that you're here!"

I looked at my mother and rolled my eyes. "Um, *I'm* Mirna. That's my mom."

"Oh . . . I'm sorry," she said, winking conspiratorially at my mother. Then she turned to me. "Hello, Mirna dear!"

After we had gone through the requisite stations—health forms, bursar, class schedule, dorm-room assignment and key, then bookstore for $300 worth of books, school supplies, and gym uniforms that we put onto my student account—we were paired with a Gold Key member who cheerfully led us through the crowds of new girls and their parents, out of Masters Hall, the main building, and up the long hill to the dorms.

I was already sweating. For reasons I can't dig far enough into my psyche to comprehend, I had dressed for the day in a green turtleneck, black pants that I had cut off at the knee, black knee-highs, and clunky black oxfords born from grunge fashion finally hitting the streets of the non-white neighborhoods of Brooklyn. The night before registration, I had stayed up late at my cousin's apartment (I was too excited to sleep anyway), letting her crimp my relaxed and shiny black hair into a style I thought appropriate for the occasion. I would be stepping into what I thought was a new identity, an unlikely boarding school student who had her own signature style (albeit borrowed from the glimpses I got from those Village folk and the hip young adults I had encountered in Park Slope).

Walking up that hill, pulling the enormous cart full of clothes and things I thought I would need, I started to worry about how I hadn't packed any T-shirts or shorts because it was supposed to be fall already. After heaving my stuff onto the old rickety elevator to the third floor, I found my room and tentatively opened the door. A thin, mousy-brown-haired girl looked up from her seat at her desk. She had been organizing her textbooks and school supplies into orderly piles, with labels and such. *She's too neat,* I thought.

"Um, hello. Are you Alana?"

"Yes, and you're Mirna, right?" she asked somewhat nervously.

"Yeah. And this is my mother, Joann."

Alana's parents, sister, and young brother were all on her side of the room; they all stopped their unpacking and turned to us.

"This is my mom, Nancy. Dad, Bernie. Brother, David, and my sister, Marah. She's a junior here."

"Hi!" We shook hands with everyone except David, who was just under five years old. He hid behind his mother.

After introductions, my mother and I started unpacking and exploring my side of the huge double room. The floors were made of polyurethane-covered cork, which I thought was fancy and reminiscent of old prewar buildings in the city.

"Girl, you have a walk-in closet. You fancy! And look at these floors! You big-time now," my mother exclaimed proudly.

There was a tall malleable lamp that would stand over the head of my bed for many a late-night reading of Fitzgerald, Knowles, Hurston, and Shakespeare. The bed was generously sized, slightly larger and longer than my twin-sized bunk bed at home, and in a wooden bed frame that put my cheap particleboard IKEA adult style to shame. The room looked over the grassy quad that was surrounded on two sides by Thompson and Cushing dorms. I would learn to love this view. In the winter, I could see all the way to the Hudson River with the Tappan Zee Bridge sparkling on cold nights.

After we had placed every piece of clothing in its proper storage space, and after my mother took away the *one* T-shirt I had thought to bring (it said "Phillips Exeter Academy," and to my mother, it would be rude of me to wear it), we made the bed. I had brought from home a black-and-red satin bedding set that looked as if it belonged more in a harem than in a ninth-grader's dorm room in Westchester County.

Meanwhile, still wearing the same clothes and dripping with sweat, my hair was becoming limp and uncrimpy. As I was rifling through my neatly folded clothing in the dresser, trying to find a more suitable shirt for the task, a tall, ruddy-faced English woman with short blond hair came into our room.

"You must be Mirna, correct? Welcome to Thompson dorm," she said with a flourish. "I'm Mrs. Hartwell, and I live downstairs on the ground floor with my family. How was your trip here?"

"It was good. We took the train."

"Oh, heavens! You must be exhausted!" She looked at me in my now-drenched turtleneck. "Do you have any T-shirts?" she asked.

"Naw, I didn't think to bring any," I said. "I thought it would be cold."

"Let me see what I have in terms of T-shirts. I'll be right back!" She hurried away and then returned. Minutes later, I had three Masters

School T-shirts that I would cherish for long after my graduation in 1993.

Soon after we finished unpacking, the dorm proctors went from door to door collecting us for the next round of orientation activities.

"Mirna? Alana? I'm Jessica, your proctor. Are you guys all set with everything?"

"I think so," I said, looking at my mother. "Ma, you ready?"

"Um, I think parents are supposed to, um, leave . . ." Jessica said, embarrassed.

"I'm gonna finish up here before I go."

We all headed down the hill to the field where we would play orientation games, and where our "big sisters" would present gift bags to us filled with Dobbs knickknacks and other important items deemed necessary for our first few weeks at the school. My big sister was Yasmeen, a tenth grader from Queens. She had long, curly extension braids and braces. We had written each other letters that summer.

"Hey, girl! Nice to finally meet you. You got everything you need?" she asked.

"Yeah, I think so." She could tell that I was nervous.

"Don't worry. You're gonna get used to all of this. I know it's a lot to take in on the first day. But in a few days you're gonna be like, what was I worried about? Promise."

I smiled and inhaled deeply. "Thanks, Yasmeen."

"Ready?" she asked, looping her elbow around mine.

"Ready."

Okay, I generally didn't enjoy having to play games in big crowds with people I didn't know, but these were fun and lighthearted, and the new girls were all just as nervous and disoriented as I was. I kept looking up out of the corner of my eye to catch quick glimpses of my mother looking down at us from the big picture window of the dining hall. After an hour or so, I became less distracted by her presence and more intertwined in the fun and anxiety down at the field. By the time we were done, I looked up at the window and she was gone.

The next stop was athletics, where both new and returning students tried out for soccer, volleyball, and field hockey. I changed into a pair of leggings and some athletic-looking shoes and headed downhill to catch a glimpse of the sports that were being offered. I was excited at the prospect of joining a team, as I had never been on one. The one-and-only team that I had ever wanted to be on was at the Philippa Duke Schuyler Middle School for the Gifted and Talented, where teachers who ran a short-lived after-school program allowed certain popular students to choose who would be on the various teams. I showed up at the hot airless gym, excited to finally be part of something at school that wasn't chorus or science club, and waited for the different interest groups to separate. Thirteen seventh-grade girls showed up, waiting patiently for the girl (probably an eighth grader) who looked like she was in charge to let us start playing. She picked five girls for one side of the net and six for the other side, leaving me leaning on the wall.

"Sorry, we don't have room for you," she'd said, turning away and walking toward the other girls. I stood there, looking awkward and feeling hurt and ashamed that I had even entertained the idea that I could be on somebody's team. I hung around for a few more minutes, hoping that a teacher or some adult figure would save me from the embarrassment and peel me off the wall. Nope. This little bitch was in charge, and I couldn't do anything about it. That had been my last flirtation with sports until the hot and humid first Saturday at Masters.

Kristina, a girl I had met that morning during registration, and I chose to go out for field hockey, after we had looked at the soccer tryouts in horror as their crazy coach, Mr. Martin, made them run ten laps just to warm up! Those girls did *not* appear to be having any fun. We definitely didn't want any part of that.

We looked at each other and made an instant and silent decision to try field hockey because we happened to be closer to the field, and the girls there didn't appear to be running much at all. *It even looks a little like golf,* I thought. *Golf doesn't look too hard, and have I ever seen golf people running on the greens?* Nope. We could definitely do this!

Neither of us knew anything about the sport or what would actually be required of us. Nevertheless, we shuffled over to the field-hockey field, which looked to be smaller than the soccer field (score!). Furthermore, the team had a woman coach who didn't look too threatening as she joked around with the returning students—those were all good signs, right?

I soon discovered how wrong I was. After running a few laps around the field (I nearly died during and after each one), we did a timed mile. What did it feel like? It felt like an asthma attack, a gunshot wound, a kick in the stomach and kidneys, slow suffocation—all topped with the whipping cream of death. I had never, ever had to run this much in one hour, let alone in one day. I had gone on long hikes with those organizations that try to turn urban kids into nature lovers (mission accomplished!), which were fairly difficult, but they had taken all day. This? This was brand-new. This was like being birthed into the world anew, like breathing for the first time and not having a clue about, well, anything.

Within the span of one short but long-feeling hour, I had to run just under a mile to warm up in order to run a mile. As I kept asking myself, *Why are we running so much?* I had a pained smile on my face. This shit was hard. I felt like death was imminent, but was so grateful to be on the field with those girls, doing what they were doing. I was simultaneously elated, scared as shit, breathless (literally), and thankful.

Before Masters, I had *no idea* what running a mile felt like because I had never had to run long for anything. The children in my neighborhood often played tag on city streets or ran races from the big, hulking gray street lamps to the alternate-side-of-street parking poles to the johnny pumps (fire hydrants), but that didn't count. We even had our own version of an obstacle course where we would line up on opposite sides of the street and hurdle or climb over each building's fences and garbage cans on the long city block. This didn't qualify as running either. None of these activities, though badass in their own right, prepared me for my first taste of long-distance running.

That first real timed mile was one of the most difficult physical things I had ever done. Also in that category was the eight-hour-long hike I did at sleep-away camp several years earlier; the climbing wall located in some woods in Milton, New Jersey; and the hike up Mount Jo in the Adirondacks with my seventh-grade classmates.

This mile consisted of two loops of the hilly campus. The start of each loop was a short but steep downhill followed by a rolling course around the storied buildings of the ninety-three-acre expanse of grassy suburban beauty. The finish of each loop was a steady uphill until it turned into one of the school's main driveways, where even the speed bumps made me tired and angry.

My mile time was around fifteen minutes—much of which I walked, huffing and puffing and nearly dying. When you have no idea what running a mile is like, or how long a mile is, and you don't have any point of reference (I would learn later that a mile is like running from your block in Brooklyn to a block in another faraway neighborhood—like running from northern Bushwick to Bed-Stuy, for example), you believe that you're going to be running and walking forever with no end to your suffering. I was disappointed to be the penultimate person, but ecstatic to not be the last.

After the mile-run debacle, practice started.

"Maybe we should have gone out for volleyball," I said, doubling over, trying to recover my breath.

"Yeah. If I'da known . . . ," Kristina responded in her thick Bronx-Italian accent.

"How was that?" Ms. Harrop asked. She was our coach, and it was apparent to all the new girls that everyone worshipped her. They all did what they were told, and didn't whine or complain about the impossible tasks placed before them.

"It was fine. It wasn't too bad. I mean, like, I could've done better," said one with a mature, husky voice and shoulder-length blond hair in tight, gelled curls.

Another girl whose legs were tan and smooth responded, "My time is slower. We were traveling all summer."

Kristina and I looked at each other, wrinkling our brows. What were they talking about? "My time is slower?" And what did she mean by "it wasn't too bad"? It was impossible. That's what it was.

"Okay, everyone line up on the hundred line," Ms. Harrop said as she ran back to the field. Were we supposed to run to the field too? I was sure Kristina and I would both be dead before the day was over.

We jogged slowly and clumsily to the field, arriving last and catching the end of Ms. Harrop's instructions.

". . . called a suicide. You'll sprint to the twenty-five-yard line, touch the paint, and sprint back."

Okay, I think I can do that.

"And then you sprint to midfield and back, the twenty-five-yard line on the other side and back, and to the other end of the field and back. Got it?"

We have to do what?

Some girls nodded their heads, ready for the challenge. Others, like Kristina and I, had dread all over our faces, like people who were about to be sentenced to death by drowning. On a basketball court, a suicide might not be so bad, but on an almost-hundred-yard-long field-hockey field, it was like someone pulling you from the sweet confines of restful death into an increasingly airless purgatory over and over again, your heart escaping from your throat and suffocating you with its explosive beating. I believe I left a lung and a half on that field.

"These will make you faster and stronger!" Ms. Harrop yelled across the field. "Field hockey is a fast game. You've gotta be able to move up and down the field quickly with no recovery. Let's go!"

While most of the girls were on their way to the hundred-yard line, I was only making it back from my seventy-five-yard sprint that wasn't a sprint anymore. To my horror, Ms. Harrop jogged up to me and paced alongside as I slowed down.

"You can do this. You did the warm-up and the mile. You can do *this*."

"But I'm slow, I can't even."

She cut me off, and I was grateful. I gasped for air.

"You'll get used to it. The first day is always the worst. I make it hard because I want to see if you're up for the challenge and if you're willing to do the work. From what I can tell, you're willing. Keep at it and finish." Then she ran down the field for a pep talk with another new girl. Did she really think I could do this? After all, I was still moving and I only had two more lengths of the field to run. I was sold. She thinks I can do this.

That practice was only the beginning of indulging in learning and growing through playing the sports of field hockey and lacrosse. That first day we sprinted lengths of the field both with and without our sticks, we practiced dribbling and driving field-hockey style, we ran some more lengths of the field, we practiced flicking the ball, and we did other activities related to field hockey. Toward the end of practice, Ms. Harrop gathered us into a circle and led us in a series of painful stretches that later on in the season would become routine and painless.

"My entire body hurts. I don't know about this." I cringed after bending forward and feeling as though the muscles in the back of my legs were about to separate from the tendons behind my knee.

"Me neither," Kristina said weakly.

"Everybody's better than us."

"Yeah, no shit. Like, all these girls have been to field-hockey camp. Um, I worked at the bowling alley with my father," she complained.

"I was in school all summer," I replied.

"I mean, did you see them running up and down the field like it wasn't a big deal? They weren't even breathing hard."

"We got a lot of work to do. Like, a lot. Are you staying?"

"Yeah, I think. You?"

"Yeah." I nodded. *Who had just taken over my brain?*

At the end of practice, we were both a sweaty mess. Never had we experienced this intensity of exercise. People did this for two and a half hours a day, five days a week? Ms. Harrop took us through what seemed like every kind of running there was—sprinting, jogging, carioca exercises, running with sticks and balls, and running backward.

———

Even after one week of practice, Kristina and I still weren't accustomed to the demands of playing a sport every day, let alone for two and a half hours each time. In fact, we were still recovering from that first day. As we started each practice, we agreed that each day we would try to do better.

As an asthmatic and someone who certainly wasn't used to running, it took a while for me to become familiar with the intensity and frequency of our daily practices after a full day of being a student at a new school.

After the first week, we hadn't yet died, so we decided that we would need to practice this other sport of running so that we wouldn't suck as much as we did at field hockey.

"We should run more," I said, one day after a grueling practice. "I'm serious. We have to get better."

Kristina looked at me, annoyed that I had suggested such a stupid thing. But she agreed.

"You're right. We're, like, the slowest ones on the team. We have to get faster. And I don't wanna suck," she said. By the end of our conversation we decided to meet up at six the next morning.

Kristina and I practiced doing the five to six loops of the field-hockey field, with its freshly cut grass and wild-onion aroma. We stopped and started, started and stopped, walked, shuffled, and bent over, breathless with chests heaving. We then made our way slowly up a humongous hill back to the dorms so we could limp into the showers before a much-welcome hot breakfast.

The earthy, pungent smell of the wild onions that grew on the sides of the old hockey field greeted us every day as we ran those warm-up loops before practice. It would always take me by surprise, causing me to wonder if they were indeed onions or if they were some unfortunate kind of wild something that no one wanted. The tall green chive-like stalks lay beneath and behind the green bench that I would spend a fair amount of time on or near during my freshman year, not playing until it was obvious that we were either winning or losing.

The field was abutted on one side by a steep hill that led to the old but stately Tudor-style dorms, and on another by a walkway and the oddly shaped 1970s / early '80s architecture of the dining hall with big picture windows that looked out every which way; on two sides, the field served as the top of a hill that led to three Cape Cod–style single-family houses hidden in a sort of cul-de-sac (if there could be one on a boarding school campus) in which dwelled the most esteemed faculty and administrators—people with power.

We ran four to six laps daily before practice to warm up before the real running began, even on the occasional Saturday when we'd have to make up a game postponed because of weather or due to having gotten lost amid the vast cemeteries of Queens. Every few weeks we ran a timed mile, and eventually my times fell from fifteen minutes to just under eleven.

Throughout the season, I grew to look forward to field-hockey practices and games. I loved the physical release of slamming our linseed-oil-slicked sticks into hard plastic balls that we sent soaring through the air, or skimming the top of the low-cut grass. Dribbling those same balls away from our opponents and returning them to the offense was satisfying in a visceral way. The game we played was hard, and in addition to skills, it required an absolute commitment to constant improvement. Our school motto was "Do It with Thy Might," and this was the expectation. In rain, extreme heat, and increasingly cold and windy days, we were to do it with our might every single day in everything that we did.

———

Ms. Harrop, our coach and athletic director, was serious about field hockey. With her, there was no whining and no pretending you were sick (because a trip to the infirmary would be worse, and you might even be given Seldane, a drug that was taken off the market a few years after I graduated); there was hard work, with the expectation of improvement and maybe a few wins, but most important, a more keenly developed athleticism.

She effortlessly and seamlessly handled both a hard plastic ball and a heavy field-hockey stick. You couldn't tell where her thin, muscular arms stopped and where the stick began. The stick was like a natural extension of her superb athleticism. The ball flew where she wished it to go, and the stick obeyed her every command whether she gripped it tightly in her hand or her fingers barely maintained contact while she extended her arm to reach a seemingly unreachable ball.

Ms. Harrop was fierce, and I wanted to be like her. I wanted to be able to run like her, easily and effortlessly while *talking* to someone, while bouncing my way up the hill to the dorms without feeling as though my heart would somehow escape my chest cavity and hurl itself through my dry, open mouth. I wanted to be able to do all that after leading a

2.5-hour-long practice and still have energy to function like a normal human being. I wanted to wake up already warmed up, with the right kind of shorts on that had the Umbro insignia on them, with a sports bra and everything, with running shoes that weren't hand-me-downs from my cousin, and finally, with a general facility about the whole business of moving without feeling as though I would keel over after every step.

Being part of a team kept us going. We knew intrinsically that if we got better, if we worked on stuff, the team would also improve. During long vacation breaks, our coaches asked us to continue running most days of the week just to stay conditioned. I took each workout seriously, planning my runs around my family's schedule and laying out my outfit the night before. I would don my best workout clothes, cotton and all. I mean, who knew? Into the front pocket of my heavy sweatshirt would go my Sony Walkman stocked with a cassette tape full of Whitney Houston, Sade, Janet Jackson, Skid Row, and Big Daddy Kane.

I would start timidly, because *no one* in my neighborhood ran just to run. People would look up at me from their stoops, before returning to what they were doing. I would run up Hart Street until it ended at a public-school track closed to the community. Then I would circle the track's perimeter and continue down my street until it ended at the Linden Hill United Methodist Cemetery. I would stop at the stone pillars at the entrance and wonder if any of the dead would mind if I ran through the paths surrounding their graves. It also gave me some pause. What if a disgruntled family member ran after me, chastising me for disturbing the dead? What if a ghost did? After a few runs, I became brazen and ran at full speed across the main path to the other side of the cemetery's boundary.

Not until I was an adult with a car did I figure out the mileage of those runs. At the most I ran two, maybe three miles. Still, it felt *epic*. I could move my body so easily along the streets where I had walked and played as a child. I was free, liberated from the gridded confines of the neighborhood. I discovered what running really was then—moving unencumbered through the world on my own two feet.

5

THE MET

The summer of 1993, the year I graduated from the Masters School, I landed a coveted high school apprenticeship at the Metropolitan Museum of Art in New York City. The application process was rather lengthy, and the day of the interview I had been suffering from the worst flu of my life.

Somehow I convinced the school nurse to release me from my quarantine in the 1970s-era infirmary to walk down the long, steep hills of Dobbs Ferry to the train station, feverish and all. I immediately passed out on the train, burning up, sweaty and chilly, and awoke to the gentle tapping of the train's conductor at Grand Central Station, the last stop. My carefully curled hair was plastered to the side of my face, and the dark skirt and thin white linen blouse I had painstakingly starched and ironed that morning were already wrinkled. I spent a few moments in the restroom before heading uptown on the subway, combing my damp, limp hair back into place, splashing cold water on my face, and straightening out my now-irretrievably rumpled outfit. *Well, I'll just have to wing it, right? It's a museum full of artists, so maybe they'll overlook my outfit. Yeah, I'll fit right in. I'm not going to worry.* I wanted to make the best impression I could, given the condition I was in. I was dizzy and light-headed, feverish, and shaky on my limbs. I managed to arrive at the interview just in time, without keeling over onto the subway tracks, and with enough medical reinforcements to help me breathe and stay alive for the next few hours.

A thin woman dressed in a short flower-print dress, opaque black tights, and thick-soled Doc Martens greeted me at the security desk in the cavernous main hall.

"Hi, Mirna. So nice to meet you! I'm Mara, the director of the Concerts and Lectures Department. We loved your application," she said as we walked toward the Egyptian Art wing. We passed a wall of hieroglyphics etched in stone with most of the beiges, browns, and brick reds weathered and faded away by age.

"Thanks! I think this would be a great opportunity to give back to the arts and learn more about arts administration and how great art institutions function." We turned into a hallway, and when she opened the first door, I was surprised to see an office. My teenage brain hadn't realized that there were actual offices in a museum. A young man with curly hair was printing tickets. A larger woman dressed in all black (jeans, T-shirt, and steel-toe Doc Martens) was on the phone with a customer who wanted to buy season tickets. Someone else was working on a concert poster that had two guitarists on it—I would later see the two brothers in concert that summer.

"As I said, we really liked what you wrote in your application about the need to have places where people can see art and create art. So why are you interested in working here? Shouldn't you be at a music camp or something?"

We continued this back-and-forth for close to forty minutes: she asked tough questions about why I thought I was qualified to work at one of the world's preeminent arts institutions, and I answered thoughtfully with what I had prepared the previous week.

"But you're a singer. What can you bring to the table as a performing artist? This is primarily a visual-arts institution," she said, perhaps expecting me to stumble. I was prepared for this.

"Well, the Met has a really successful concert hall. I was actually here for a violin concert a few weeks ago. Up until then, I didn't even know there was a theater here. I think everyone should know about this place, that they can come and look at Greek sculptures and Egyptian hieroglyphics and then go to a concert with top-notch performers afterwards. I mean, that's pretty cool."

I managed to remain upright throughout the entire interview, although I could feel the meds wearing off. I didn't sweat or tremble, and if the woman could tell I was sick, she didn't let on.

———

A few days later, I got the position, a dream job for someone who had begun to seriously consider a life in the arts (no matter which arts they were). I headed to work eagerly every day.

I started in the Concerts and Lectures Department and was responsible for easy tasks like mailing tickets, communicating with ticket holders, and resolving issues as they came up.

"Mirna, can you come over here a minute?" Mara asked one day after I had worked there a few weeks.

"I have an idea. I think the ticket stuff is probably boring for you, so how about we do some special projects?"

"Like what?" I asked. "I mean, I'd love to, whatever it is."

"I'd like you to do some research on other venues, like the 92nd Street Y, Alice Tully Hall, and Symphony Space. Also, see what's going on downtown in similar-sized venues. Look at their schedules, see who's performing and when, get a sense of the variety . . . Is it mostly classical, folk, or jazz? What are they playing? New music? Traditional? What's the caliber of the performers? Are they well known or early career? Find out everything. Make a calendar with all your findings. And then you'll present your findings to us in a few weeks. You up for it?" Mara said, barely looking at me.

"On it!"

My new project required research, scheduling appointments with venue managers, coming up with ideas for future concerts and lectures based on what was lacking at other venues, attending and ushering various concerts at the museum (the double-guitar concert with the Assad Brothers was my favorite!), helping to write and edit concert notes, and performing other tasks that catapulted my learning and expertise in the classical-music concert scene of New York City.

The other part of the job that I enjoyed was the requirement for all summer apprentices to "fulfill" time perusing the works at the museum each day and report on our findings to our supervisors. I spent many hours in the Islamic Art wing admiring intricate mosaic tile work and calligraphy, and in American Furniture, marveling the plain beauty of Shaker handiwork. However, I spent the bulk of my time immersed in the grandeur of the Temple of Dendur and its adjacent garden. The job was perfect. I could commute to Manhattan from Brooklyn, which was still an enjoyable novelty at the time, and work at a prestigious historical institution with prestigious people and prestigious, highfalutin art.

The Met is situated on the northeastern edge of Central Park, a mecca for all things urban outdoors, a perfect location for an aspiring in-line skater like myself. Each day I would walk from the Eighty-Sixth Street subway station and long to be one of the runners or in-line skaters I could see from Fifth Avenue engrossed in the physicality of their activities. I decided that I wanted to be one of them. I wanted to look graceful on a slick pair of wheels. It was almost as though it were a more elevated level of the skating I had done on Hart Street. On traditional roller skates I could move forward and backward and weave my legs in and out. But in-line skating was a different beast, and learning how to do it well would mean that I had reached another level in my physical sophistication.

A friend of mine from high school had given me a pair of in-line skates as an end-of-year present (she had also purchased a pair for herself and was hoping I would join her on our hilly school campus), so I was determined to skate. The in-line skates were heavy, cumbersome, and difficult to put on, and remove, especially from sweaty feet. But I was determined. I bought a set of kneepads and wrist guards with my first check and carried the whole kit in my backpack to work, the entire time trying to look like a pro. I tied the skates together by the laces and threw them over my shoulders. On the subway, they were unwieldy as they sat between my feet, as they kept rolling forward and then falling sideways. Yeah, I looked the expert.

I tried to hold in my excitement as the day progressed. I pictured myself gliding effortlessly on Park Drive along with everyone else after work. I already had it planned out. I'd make it look easy, flawless. I'd do tricks, such as squatting on one leg like I could do in regular skates. I'd go backward and then easily pivot in the other direction without ever losing balance. I couldn't wait!

After work I headed straight to the nearest park entrance and sat on a bench to put on my skates. I had actually done a tiny bit of in-line skating on my block in Brooklyn for practice, so I knew I was ready.

I don't know if it was the knowledge that much-more-expert folks would be out there skating and watching my clumsy ass, or if it was a fear of falling, but I was suddenly concerned about what other folks would think of me on these big-ass skates. I was petrified, not of falling itself, but of falling in front of other people, of losing my balance, and of looking like an unwieldy dork.

I kind of looked the part; now I needed to *be* the part. I stood up on wobbly legs and struggled to catch my balance. *A-ha!* It's the stupid backpack—a green JanSport that had been all the rage that year. I hadn't skated with it before and so it threw off my balance, just enough that

I immediately bent over and was barely able to control any sudden forward motion.

I managed to somehow get upright and continue forward, although still on wobbly legs. I was moving, though, and soon started feeling more at home on the skates. I practiced some moves: stopping using the heel brake (which is different from traditional skating), weaving my feet in and out, skating upright and in a bent position like I'd seen countless ice-skaters do on TV, complete with my hands behind my back and making some turns. I was hot and sold.

For the next few days, I skated on and off, but ultimately I decided that the skates were too big of a commitment to bring to work every day. Hence, the next obvious option was to join the runners. Heck, I'd already been running for four years now, so all I needed were the right shoes to look and be just like the other runners.

I felt empowered: I would become a *runner in Central Park*, like those folks who ran in groups small and large, individually, or with large, clunky jogging strollers carrying sleeping children. They strode gracefully, with earphones on their heads attached to Discmen and fashionable, haute couture running clothes—loose shorts and close-fitting singlets. Sweaty and determined, they ran Park Drive and the bridle trails that always seemed to lead to nowhere. I wanted to be like them: runnerly and fit, carefree, laser-focused, and light on my feet.

I often passed a shoe store on my walks back and forth to lunching at the Papaya King. The store was actually more like a variety shop, where high-heeled fashion boots, steel-toe work boots, and sneakers shared the same wall space. I walked in and two sales associates immediately greeted me, probably because they thought I had come in to steal something.

"I'm looking for a pair of running shoes," I said.

One of them, a young man who looked to be in his early twenties, stepped forward to help me.

"You got any in size 11?" I asked, already guessing what his answer might be.

"I don't think we carry that size," he replied.

"Can you at least check?"

After some annoyed hesitation, the surly jerk rolled his eyes. "Yeah, hold on."

As I waited for him to bring me a suitable pair of shoes that fit, I hoped this wouldn't be like every other store that didn't carry women's shoes larger than a size 10. I worried that I would have to leave, shoeless and embarrassed to have been born with square-shaped Flintstones feet.

"I *actually* found something," he said, returning with two boxes. The first was a pair of forest-green Adidas. The other was a pair of a brand I had never heard of (Brooks) with an insignia that certainly wasn't as cool or as ubiquitous as the Nike swoosh or the three Adidas stripes. I had no intention of wearing a wannabe brand that looked as if they could be sold at Payless. Furthermore, they cost upward of seventy dollars, and with my small check of $200, I wouldn't have been able to afford them anyway.

"I'll try on the Adidas pair," I said. They cost a mere thirty-five bucks, so I'd still be able to afford lunch from Papaya King for a few days plus buy an article of clothing at the Gap, contribute to a few meals at home, pay for my own transportation to and from work, and buy a one-way Amtrak ticket to Elyria, Ohio, the town closest to Oberlin, where I would be heading to college in August.

As I tried them on, I marveled at how well they fit and the fact that they would be the first real running shoes that I had bought with my own money.

"How many miles do you run on a daily basis?" the sales associate asked.

"Um, I don't know, one or two," I answered.

The dude snickered and shook his head almost imperceptibly.

"Can I just buy the shoes, please?" *Jesus.* I'm not sure what inspired him to exhibit such assholery, but I was undeterred. I needed the shoes for my next adventure in Central Park.

After paying, I exited the store. That small interaction with the jerk tainted my afternoon a little, but I didn't let him dampen my desire to become one of those fluid beings in the park.

The next day I began running in the park, which was way easier than skating. I didn't have a learning curve, except now I'd be surrounded by people who took running so seriously you could see it in their faces—how they furrowed their brows while moving; how they became annoyed when tourists crossed in front of them, slowing their pace; how they seemed simultaneously ecstatic and pain ridden. I was a slow runner among these gazelles, but I didn't care. All that mattered was that I was also taking part in the sport, in beautiful Central Park.

Running in Central Park and on Hart Street, I felt alive and athletic. I laced up my kicks and headed out in the rain, in the heat, on perfectly gorgeous days, in my own neighborhood in Brooklyn, at school outside of lacrosse and field-hockey practice, during my summer music program at Skidmore, and later during my semester abroad in Spain while I was a student at Oberlin. Even though I didn't consider myself a real runner, I ran or jogged as much as I could—and I was developing runner habits. Those few miles set the tone for the day, and would later set the tone for my life as an adult.

6

THE UNBEARABLE LIGHTNESS OF RUNNING

Three grapefruits escaped from the flimsy plastic bag between my feet and rolled across the dirty floor of the subway car as the train lurched forward, leaving the dank and humid Ninety-Sixth Street station. I jumped up to save the fruit that I had purchased at Fairway Market from certain death, trying to impress my newish boyfriend with my high level of New Yorker sophistication. I used extra-virgin olive oil, the kind that would cloud up because it was so pure, so unadulterated by canola and vegetable oil, so authentic and so, so not Goya or Bertolli. I bought organic wine from the Union Square Greenmarket and bagels from H&H. I dined at Dan Tempura near Sixty-Eighth and at Nascimento on First. I spent weekends rifling through used books on the Upper West Side after I had eaten *feijoada* at the Coffee Shop in Union Square, admiring all the sexy servers pandering strong coffee, caipirinha shooters, and plantains. I stopped at the HMV to purchase the newest remastering of classical symphonies and opera, chamber music, and Beethoven sonatas. I spent many hours at Starbucks poring over the *Times*, devouring every article in the magazine like a hungry child, eagerly anticipating the moment when I would turn the page to the Sunday crossword that I would start at the café, continue on the train (making sure no wandering eyes watched my vocabulary mis-steps), and finish at home with the help of a still-young Internet.

Cito didn't care for any of it. His dark-brown eyes had pleaded with me for months to allow him to accompany me to my apartment in Riverdale. For months I had hugged and kissed him, then bid him adieu at whatever subway station we ended up at after our weekly Tuesday date—he would stand forlornly at the top of the steps while I bounded downstairs as quickly as possible to protect *myself* from giving in and inviting him over.

Cito was gentle and kind. He worked long hours pumping gas in New Jersey, making two to three dollars per hour, but he always insisted that he pay for dinner. Everywhere we went, and I often picked the res-taurant, he sipped on tea or slurped on a bowl of soup. I ordered with abandon—dragon rolls from my favorite sushi shop Dan Tempura on the Upper West Side, *chapchae* from Wonjo in Koreatown, or *pierogis* and borscht from Veselka on the Lower East Side. I wanted to show him the world through food, and he wished to show me his heart by emptying his wallet and indulging my eclectic appetite.

He spoke in a halting but musical English, accented by both a West African Francophone French and his tribal language, Moré. When he spoke on his cell phone to his family and friends, his voice would rise and fall excitedly, the conversation punctuated by laughter and sounds of disbelief.

"*Eh! Manawana!*" he would exclaim, greeting whomever had called. I would listen patiently, trying to figure out the French parts of the conversation.

"*Ça va? . . . Oui, ça va. Je suis à New York avec ma biche.*"

Ma biche? What the hell? I am no one's bitch! I soon figured out that it was slang for girlfriend or honey.

He continued, "*Et chez toi? Ça va?*"—this back-and-forth, asking how the family was and then how individual people were doing, lasted a few minutes. I didn't understand why there was so much asking after people before an actual conversation happened.

On all of our dates, we ate (I drank liquor and he sipped more tea) and walked around whatever neighborhood of Manhattan we were in. When it was time for me to head back home, I was firm and unrelenting.

"No, you can't come over. I . . . can't." I was falling for him so hard; I was frightened of the prospect of loving him deeply. I knew that if he came over, there would be no turning back. I wasn't ready to take this step.

———

That night on the Bronx-bound 1 train with the grapefruits was different, however.

It was mid-May of 1999 when we had met up outside the Hospital for Special Surgery, where I had just finished my weekly Tuesday Avon Mini Marathon training program. Running was difficult that warm and humid April evening. The organizers of the training program had enlisted the help of several professional athletes to lead different pace groups. I was paired with Marla Thomas, an Olympic-level track-and-field athlete who helped me run four miles without stopping for the first time ever.

The day's workout had been the most rewarding but challenging of them all. We had started out with a half mile of warm-ups running the esplanade to a big hill. We stretched, both statically and dynamically, and then were split up into pace groups. I'm not sure if the leaders were tired of me running so slowly, or if they believed that I had the potential to run stronger than I had been (I choose to believe the latter), so I was in a pace group of my own with Marla.

"I heard you been killin' it out here," she said, after she introduced herself and shook my hand. I was surprised by how firm it was. "They said you're ready to run without stopping."

"For real? They said that?" I asked, incredulous. "I don't—I don't think . . ."

"Sure you can. That's why I'm here, to help you with that. You ready?" she asked while stretching her quads.

This woman with her '90s version of the '80s Jheri curl, the Wave Nouveau, was dark-skinned like me with an imposing stature and exuded an air of quiet but authoritative strength. She didn't look like what I imagined an Olympic-level athlete would look like, with her tracksuit pants and plain white T-shirt, but her defined, muscular arms told a different story.

"I guess I don't have a choice, do I?"

"Not really." She cocked her head and flashed a brilliant smile. "Let's go, sis."

We headed north on the East Side Esplanade. Marla ran about two feet ahead of me for the first mile. I kept her pace, having a hard time of it in the beginning. My breathing eventually evened out, as did my strides. We ran in silence until we arrived at a concrete staircase.

"Oh boy," I said between breaths.

"You can do it. Don't think about it. Land on the top half of your feet, almost on your toes. Swing your arms."

I dug deep and made an effort to bounce lightly up the stairs. It was difficult, but not astonishingly so. When we got to the top, she continued running.

"Marla, I think I need to take a break . . . ," I pleaded.

"No, you don't." She kept running. I followed.

Two miles in we turned around. My legs were now warm, and although the pace was fast for me, I was able to keep up with a real athlete, who was probably struggling with running at such a slow pace. But I forgot all about that. I stopped thinking about how difficult it was to run at this pace. I started to notice all the runners and walkers out on this early-spring night. I listened to the sounds of a city slowing down almost imperceptibly.

Three miles. Almost there . . .

I ran into the light, slightly fishy breeze coming off the East River. I watched cars traveling back and forth from Queens on the Fifty-Ninth Street Bridge and, just beyond, a flash of red where the Tram carried passengers from Manhattan to Roosevelt Island.

"You doin' it!" Marla cheered from behind. At some point during the final mile, she decided to hang back and let me take the lead. Surprisingly, I ran the entire time, without stopping. Since finishing high school, my running routine had included sporadic bursts of running, but I always used a run/walk method. I could run a mile or two without stopping, but three? Four? This was new territory.

A quarter of a mile from the end of our run, I felt a familiar twinge in the corners of my eyes. There was a small group of other participants and coaches waiting for Marla and me at the finish.

I dug deep and sped up.

"Let's get this done!" Marla called from behind. "Go, girl!"

I felt weightless as I sailed into an improvised chute of people who high-fived me as I finished my run. They enveloped my heaving, sweaty body in an equally sweaty group hug. I cried.

Marla came over and shook my hand again. This time she followed that with a hug.

"You see? You did it. I told you. Never, ever doubt yourself. Never."

"Thank you, Marla. Thank you for running with me. I'm sorry I—"

"Stop. You did a great job out there. I knew you could do it. You're ready for that 10K. You've been ready, but now you actually know."

I had found the ad for the running clinic while flipping through my daily dosage of the *New York Times* during a break at my desk in my corner cubby on the sixteenth floor of a nondescript office building in Newark, New Jersey. Just a few weeks before, I had joined the office gym with a work friend and set out to get back into some sort of physical routine. Since graduating from college in December of 1997, I was preoccupied with finding a job that could possibly lead to either a financial or legal career in corporate America. I worked as a paralegal, a consultant, and a legal translator all while working at Starbucks evenings and weekends, continuing to study voice with a consortium of teachers in New York City, coaching opera roles, auditioning, and performing monthly with a small group of opera singers. I had also gained some weight, my paycheck providing almost unlimited access to high-end-restaurant meals and my newest predilection, Spanish red wine.

Reentering my family's home life and routines in Brooklyn was difficult. I had lived away from home since my freshman year in high school, and having to abide by rules dictated by the presence of children and teenagers still at home was odd and discomforting. The minute I returned home in the middle of the school year—I graduated a semester early from my double-degree program—I started looking for a job. The search took over my life, my resources, and any time I would have normally devoted to my physical fitness routine. Sending résumés, answering ads, visiting temp agencies, taking typing and personality tests, and being interviewed by some of the shrewdest businessmen and women in New York City at companies and firms like Morgan Stanley Dean Witter, Sullivan and Cromwell, Citibank, and Credit Suisse became part of my daily rhythm.

I found a home within a series of paralegal temporary positions, learning what I could about corporate and litigation law. I earned good money and was eventually able to move out of my childhood home into my own one-bedroom apartment in the leafy Riverdale neighborhood of the Bronx. After temping for a few months, a friend mentioned my name to some project managers at the consulting firm KPMG. I set up an interview and was immediately hired for a big on-site project in Newark, New Jersey—a ninety-minute commute by train from my new place.

My job involved poring over details of clients' medical records, actuarial information used in deciding insurance worthiness, and snippets of conversations between agents and the insured. I was quick and accurate and learned the language of insurance so well that I surprised an insurance agent who had come to my house for an initial consult.

Mr. Higginbottom was his name, a gentleman from South Carolina who was about to retire. He came to my apartment on a Saturday morning, dressed in an immaculate gray suit. His shoes had been shined recently, and his briefcase smelled of weathered leather.

"So, Miss Valerio, what are you looking for in an insurance policy? You seem young and healthy. But you never know what'll happen the next hour or the next day. You want to be prepared, leave something for your funeral expenses."

He continued in his southern, low country accent. "Now would be a great time to start paying on a policy—"

"What do you think of variable annuities?" I interrupted. "I mean, I'm trying to decide between a VAL and traditional whole life. Part of me wants to risk the volatility of the stock market, but the other part of me wants to be more conservative." I was showing off.

"Where did you say you worked again?" Mr. Higginbottom asked, confused.

"Oh, I work as a consultant."

Still stumped, he asked, "What else do you know?"

"Look, I don't want to get screwed over by someone trying to sell me a policy I don't want or need, not that you would do that."

"Okay then, Miss Valerio. You seem like you know what you're talking about." I smiled, proud of myself.

"I'd like a fifty thousand dollar whole-life policy, please."

———

A major storm hit the city in the midwinter of 1999. Some friends had notified me that both Penn Stations in Newark and Manhattan had lost power because of the ice and winds from the storm and that I was probably going to be stuck at work at KPMG for the foreseeable future. All

PATH trains had also stopped running. I didn't have any close friends in the office at that point, and I needed some overtime, so I decided to chill, work, and wait it out.

At about nine in the evening, word got around that both stations were up and running. I gathered my stuff and hurried down to the lobby so that I could make the first PATH train back to the World Trade Center. I was tired, hungry, and annoyed that I was the only person left at work—in this nondescript, personality-free, cubicle-filled, blue-industrial-carpet-laden building.

After I paid my fare, I walked onto the cold and windy platform. I was wearing a heavy, down-filled green Eddie Bauer jacket with thick woolen mittens that were the only gift my parents could afford to give me for Christmas freshman year in college. With my mittened hand, I carried a thin plastic bag that held the remains of my home-cooked lunch in several disposable bowls. I also had a huge but soft leather bag on my shoulder that contained several books, including Milan Kundera's *The Unbearable Lightness of Being* and Umberto Eco's *Travels in Hyperreality*; that day's *New York Times* crossword; an assortment of pens, pencils, and markers; and a wallet stuffed to the brim with things I didn't need, such as coffee receipts, old college IDs, an expired Ohio learner's permit, and several business cards whose owners and occasions for meeting I couldn't remember.

To top it off, I wore a warm but misshapen woolen cap. At this point in my life, I didn't care how I looked. In fact, I never cared how I looked, which always seemed the condition I was in when various folks wanted to strike up a conversation.

As I stood on the PATH train platform, a tall man in a blue, puffy triple-goose-down jacket and tight beanie on his oval-shaped head walked toward me, gave me a slightly leering once-over, and headed further down the platform.

I was becoming more and more annoyed after waiting at least fifteen minutes. At this rate, I'd get home late and sleep only a few hours before having to return to work for another long day that started at seven. I was cranky and tired and *not* in the mood for being checked out.

I turned my body away so that I wouldn't catch his eye.

After a few more minutes of waiting for the train that wouldn't come, I saw this guy heading toward me out of the corner of my eye. *Oh Jesus, really? Not tonight.*

"Eh, excuse me? Miss?" he stammered in a halting and thickly accented English.

"Yeah?" I said, my eyebrows raised and full New York armor deployed.

"Eh, please can you tell me which train this is?"

"It's the train to New York," I said bluntly, pointing to a nearby sign.

"Thanks, miss."

"Yep."

Oh, okay . . . he only wanted to ask a question.

Relieved that this guy wasn't trying to "talk" to me, I returned to my angry and impatient pondering of the train situation.

Some minutes later, he approached me again, this time with a different question.

"Um, if I'm gonna go to Brooklyn, which station do I need get off?" he asked.

"Last stop," I said. He'd better not come at me again with another stupid question.

The train finally came into the station after we had waited for almost an hour on the platform and after I had been peppered with several more questions about how he could get to Brooklyn. Before it came to a stop, he approached me yet again.

"Which car should I sit in?" he asked.

I looked at him like anyone who grew up in Brooklyn might look at a tourist family standing in the middle of Broadway, maps open.

"Doesn't matter," I said curtly.

I entered the train, and he took this opportunity to sit in the same car, plopping down several seats away from me and bobbing his head to some radio station he had playing in his head. I turned away, dug out the Kundera, and started hate-reading it. I despised the book from the first page, but unfortunately I was at a point in my life in which finishing what I started reading was an absolute necessity. I've become wiser since then.

I read, hating the misogynistically imagined characters—the dog, even. But I kept reading, if only to help ignore this guy who was now staring at me quite openly and unabashedly.

After a few minutes had transpired, this man, who couldn't have been more than twenty-five, began to sidle his way over to me (the train was nearly empty, facilitating his deft move).

"What are you reading?" he asked.

"A book."

"I know but, eh, which?"

Like you'll know, I thought.

"It's by Milan Kundera." I was sure that answer would leave him puzzled and possibly turned off by my eclectic reading tastes.

"Oh, yes of course!" he exclaimed, becoming excited. "The Czech author. Yes! He wrote *The Book of Laughter and Forgetting!* Yes, I know his books!"

This man who had been longing for my attention had placed himself in quite the desirable position. He was obviously a Reader, with a capital *R*, because seriously, who reads Kundera and is actually inspired to read more than one of his works of fiction? Yeah, like nobody I knew, except for those who enjoyed postmodernism, and those weren't any of *my* friends.

I stared for a long time, puzzled, because I hadn't had a conversation about books with an actual guy in ages. Or maybe never. I'm going to go with never.

"Come again? You know about Milan Kundera?" I asked.

My eyes lit up at the mention of another book, and I was speechless for a couple of seconds, reconsidering my initial impression of this foreign guy who sported a wide gap between his two front teeth.

"You have read Chinua Achebe? *Things Fall Apart*? Yes? And *Arrow of God*? Yes?"

Now *I* felt like an idiot. I had *Things Fall Apart* on my bookshelf, but had I read it? *No.* And *Arrow of God* I hadn't read either.

This dude was playing me at my own game. I usually gave this type of unspoken quiz to the three whole guys who had attempted courting me: Oh, you're a computer programmer? Have you read any Calvino? Oh, you're an MBA and we work the same job that I got with my lowly BA? Have you read any bell hooks? Any García Márquez? Do you like poetry? Do you listen to classical music? Museums, do you even go to museums? Concerts? Do you listen to jazz?

I was relentless and unsatisfied with the slim pickings that the dating world offered for an educated black woman college graduate. Hence, my guard was always up. I shunned anyone who gave even the slightest hint that he didn't appreciate having or seeking knowledge and living a life of intellectual curiosity, like Winston Carrington, the skinny Jamaican guy who kept his apartment heated like a Caribbean beach, but perhaps more importantly had questioned my desire to continue singing classical music and asked me what my real job was going to be in the future.

After I retrieved my grapefruits from under someone else's legs, I slid back into my seat next to Cito, who had agreed to run with me in the morning even though he had no athletic clothing with him, including sneakers. I was due to run a total of forty minutes, alternating running and walking in intervals of ten minutes of running to two minutes of walking. I had become serious about training at six most mornings on both the crushed-cinder pathway of Van Cortlandt Park and its more secluded trails. I wasn't about to deviate from my schedule because some skinny African guy who could barely speak English was coming over to my small fourth-floor apartment. I would run the next day, even if I had to kick him out in the morning.

"You can sleep here," I said, bringing him a comforter from my bedroom, avoiding eye contact. "Do you want me to pull out the sofa? It's really comfortable."

He pulled me close to him and lifted my chin. "I'm sleeping in there, with you. Okay?" His eyes offered no choice.

We awoke the next morning, entangled and spent. I couldn't imagine getting out of bed, running and acting as though things hadn't changed drastically. I had just slept with this man. We had crossed my carefully constructed boundary. Moreover, my morning routine had been disrupted. I was supposed to be outside running, yet I remained wrapped in his arms, eyes wide open and mind racing.

"You have to go. I'm sorry, I can't do this. I . . . I can't." I freed myself from his arms. They smelled faintly of expensive cologne and lotion.

"What happened? I did something wrong?" he asked, confused. And hurt.

"No, just, I can't. You just gotta go. I'm sorry. I'm so sorry. Please . . ."

He arose from the bed silently and began to dress. I took the opportunity to go to the bathroom. I couldn't look at him; I was so conflicted and embarrassed by my odd behavior. I looked in the mirror and mouthed, *What the fuck is wrong with you, Mirna? What did you just do?*

I returned to the bedroom while he gathered his things in the living room. I still couldn't look at him.

"Okay . . . I'm gonna, I'm gonna go. I—"

"Um, I'm so sorry. I'm . . ."

"It's okay. I'll see you. I love you." Cito pulled me into his blue jacket and kissed me. I inhaled deeply to remember his scent. I was sure I had hurt him so much that I wouldn't ever see him again.

We walked to the door and I opened it, moving aside so he could leave. I watched him as he walked down the steps. Then I ran to my window and watched him leave the courtyard painted red. I plopped on the sofa and lay there for a bit, staring at the ceiling.

When I finally summoned the courage to get up from the couch (and call in sick to work), out of the corner of my eye I spotted a yellow sticky note on the wall next to the door.

C. A. R. N.

His full initials, written in big, sprawling, and curly formal handwriting.

I love you!

Fortunately, for me, Cito recovered fairly quickly from my awkwardness. He called that evening after work and asked me how I was doing without nary a mention of that morning and previous evening. We reconnected the following week. I went for a run on Wednesday morning without him, and fourteen months later we were married.

7

THE IRONY OF LEHIGH VALLEY

While still living in the Riverdale neighborhood of the Bronx, Cito, Rashid (even though he was still a baby), and I led active if somewhat chaotic lives. We lived in a fourth-floor walk-up in a just-starting-to-decay prewar building, which of course meant it had lots of character and characters. One woman lived in the building with her eight children. Another resident suffered from paranoid schizophrenia and was a hoarder. A violinist and music therapist who was dating a jazz trumpeter who happened to have been a friend from college lived on the top floor of the building. Two jazz musicians lived to the left of us, one another trumpeter who looked and played startlingly like Miles Davis. The other was a balding white guy in his midforties who played an excellent and sultry alto saxophone. They once got into a heated argument about rent that involved crashing and smashing various items in their apartment (we could hear *everything* through the walls). One of them pulled out a gun and then the police arrived. A few days later, both were gone.

Jerome and his Filipina wife, Myrna, lived on the bottom floor. He was a New York City taxicab driver and a wildly talented violinist and pianist, who I would see talking to no one in particular as he went about his daily routine. Sometimes I'd hear long, beautiful violin cadenzas or Brahms piano music flowing from his apartment window.

One day I was practicing "Come scoglio" from Mozart's opera *Così fan tutte* for an upcoming concert with Intercambio Musicale, my operatic performance group. I heard a hard and impatient knock on my door.

I looked through the peephole, saw Jerome, and immediately opened the door.

"Was that you singing and, um, playing?" he asked.

"Yeah . . . ," I answered, not knowing what he was getting at. "Come in." He walked in and made a beeline for my Hardman and Peck baby grand.

"Wow! Nice instrument. This yours?"

"Um, yeah . . . I bought it last year."

"Oh nice, a solid American make—good bones. Um . . . can I play for you? I love *Così*."

Jerome sat down on the bench, did a few scales to test the weight and action of the keys, and looked up. "Really nice. You ready?"

"Let's do it!"

Jerome played the opening chords with fervor, and I imitated his energy. I had never sung the aria in quite that way. I also hadn't witnessed anyone sight-read music as perfectly as he did since my days at Oberlin. I was impressed and overjoyed to be making music with such a phenomenal musician.

"Wow! I've been meaning to come up here for a while. I love your voice. I love hearing you sing. You know, I can hear you sometimes when I'm taking a walk in Van Cortlandt Park."

"Really?" I asked, a bit incredulous.

"Yeah. Like when you sing Rachmaninoff, I can hear you. Are you studying? Auditioning? Where are you performing again?"

I loved so much about that building. People like me, like us—musicians, writers, college students, young professionals just starting families and learning how to balance careers with the demands of children and spouses—filled its quirky, parquet-floored, white-walled prewar apartments. The neighborhood was beautiful and convenient to both Manhattan and Westchester County. Van Cortlandt Park—one of New York City's gems of green space with beautiful trails, fields, bodies of water, and a public golf course—was just a few hundred feet away.

I went up and down the stairs running errands, walking to and from the supermarket eleven blocks away, and carrying dozens of heavy bags of groceries. After Rashid was born, I carried him up and down the four flights of stairs in a fully loaded Peg Perego stroller, with a diaper bag and an assortment of reading materials, such as the *New York Times*, crosswords, an irreverent parenting book or two, and a journal for jotting down thoughts, so I could read both to me and him on the train, and other things we might need—you know, just in case.

Rashid and I traveled everywhere together, even if it meant breaking down his heavy stroller and maneuvering various bags and other sundries—all in one fell swoop—as the shuttle bus came (because the L train never ran when you needed it to), getting on the bus, hoping someone would at least give us space in the crowd, and doing it all over again, day after day. The rare times I did leave the house alone, I made sure to go to the gym. Other times, Rashid and I went to the 92nd Street Y for family swim. (I was determined to raise a swimmer, especially as a black parent, because I didn't want my son to be another drowning statistic of black and Hispanic people who don't know how to swim.)

As Rashid grew and became a bit heavier, I started carrying him in an unwieldy Kelty backpack that garnered lots of curious stares, even in New York. I also was determined not to give in to the little bit of postpartum blues, so I kept moving and made sure I was busy.

Free kids' activity at some park in another borough? We were there.

Beach? There.

Trip to Nice, France, so Mom could participate in a master class with her former Juilliard voice teacher? Yes, there too.

My mostly childless friends were particularly endearing. If any of them felt like I was spending too much time indoors, they came over and retrieved me, taking me on hikes in Bear Mountain and long walks in Van Cortlandt Park so that I'd have someone to interact with who wasn't my husband or child.

"I'm coming over, and we're going to take a walk," said David, a friend from college who happened to live a few blocks away.

"I'm fine, I think. I'm just overwhelmed."

"Well, I'm coming over anyway. You need to get out of that apartment."

A few miles, conversations, and raindrops later, I came home rejuvenated and ready to deal with more baby stuff.

———

I was purposefully active during my pregnancy. I wanted to make sure that I did my best to avoid those risks I thought I could prevent or at least slow down, such as gestational diabetes, preeclampsia, extra weight on my already overtaxed frame, and cankles, because that's what all the activity was really about. I was dead set on avoiding cankles in every possible way. I knew intellectually that the body does what it wants and what it needs, but I was hoping fervently to have some say in this particular issue. I walked a lot. Even though I knew I'd have to use the bathroom about a hundred times a day, I drank a lot of water to stay hydrated. I swam at my gym a few times a week. I disembarked from the subway train at a station forty to sixty blocks from where I needed to be, just to walk some extra miles. I purchased a bunch of yoga-for-pregnancy videos and did them religiously, every morning before work. I squatted, a lot. I squatted so much that my mother-in-law worried I was going to hurt myself.

Many days I ran and walked in the park, walked to the Bally's gym and worked out, and explored the hills of Riverdale. I've always been the peripatetic type—much like the Energizer Bunny, going and going and going, wandering anywhere and everywhere on foot.

In fact, the day before Rashid was born, I had my final prenatal doctor's appointment, visited my mother at the coffee shop where she worked, finished the book I was reading (something about a mean magazine editor who terrorized her underlings for the sake of art), rode the train home to the Bronx, and was still antsy. I took my mother-in-law, Fatimata, on a three-hour hike in Van Cortlandt Park along the Aqueduct and John Muir Trails. Later that evening, I danced for a few hours at my ten-year high school reunion and drank a glass of chilly white wine. This child was already a week past the due date; I needed for this baby to not be snuggling atop my bladder and resting his long feet on my right rib.

Two days prior, my mother-in-law and I had been running errands, trying to be as prepared as we could—the bag for the hospital was already packed. (Nota bene: you can never really be fully prepared for a child's arrival, for said child will come with his or her own schedule and doesn't give a damn about the plans you made in your uninitiated-parent mind.) Fatimata and I had spent time squatting and lifting, putting Rashid's fancy Italian crib together (the crib that he would sleep in for a total of about ten hours over the course of a year, and I'm probably overestimating here). We walked up and down the stairs visiting the corner bodegas, buying last-minute items like baby laundry detergent because we needed it *right now*. I moved my bedroom around, again, ensuring that there would be sufficient space for egress in case of a fire. Eventually I moved all of the furniture back into its original arrangement.

Rashid was born the day after the hike and the party. The contractions started soon after Fatimata and I returned from our evening out. They weren't painful at first. In fact, they felt similar to the periodic Braxton-Hicks contractions I had experienced throughout the last three months of the pregnancy. I slept fitfully, making several trips to the bathroom until I didn't make it. My water finally broke in the small passageway between my bedroom and the bathroom during one of these trips, gushing what seemed like gallons of warm fluid onto the hallway floor. At around five in the morning we jumped into a cab and headed to Lenox Hill Hospital in Manhattan.

At exactly 4:00 p.m., the resident in charge was ready for me to start pushing. I didn't feel any pain after the epidural had been administered, but couldn't ignore the intense pressure of the increasingly rhythmic contractions. This child was ready to be born.

I pushed for fifty minutes, in front of a rapt audience that included the resident (my obstetrician was at his brother's college graduation), an intern, my mother, Cito's mother, and a sweating, hyperventilating husband. We returned home to the Bronx two days later, Rashid and I both a little sore and beat up, but healthy. After recuperating a bit, I slowly returned to my daily rhythm, running errands, making my best attempt to live the life of an active mom with newborn baby in tow.

I know of no yoga pose called Downward Dog with Child, but Rashid must have known something that I didn't. In fact, I think he had extrasensory perception and other superpowers when he was around eighteen months. Every morning I silently slipped out of bed at around four o'clock onto our carpeted floor, praying that my movements hadn't jostled him awake. I tiptoed soundlessly to the kitchen like the Brooklyn ninja I was, brewed a cup of coffee to help wake both body and mind, and laid down my sticky yoga mat for my daily getting-to-know-my-body-again practice.

Rashid had different plans, however. As I started easing my tight back into a forward bend, he would toddle into the living room and crawl under me the moment I moved into Downward Dog. He would sit there, cross-legged and silent, until I eventually had to move out of the pose for fear my trembling arms would crumble and force my heavy body atop his not-yet-two-year-old body.

He would have *none* of this whole mommy-time business, and the idea of weaning from nursing was hilarious to him. His ritual of calmly waiting for me to be done while obstructing any further movement was his way of reminding me that I now had someone else to prioritize. Like many women, I suffered from sleep deprivation as soon as he was born. I nursed Rashid on call, and even though I eventually mixed in prepared formula so that he would sleep longer and deeper, he still had trouble sleeping for more than two hours at a time.

———

In 2004, when Rashid was a little more than a year old, we moved to Owings Mills, Maryland, to one of those overly planned multifunction business/residential communities where identical rows of hastily constructed townhomes surrounded what was supposed to have been the lifeblood of this Baltimore suburb.

After having pieced together a series of part-time gigs soon after Rashid was born, the Park School of Baltimore, one of the premier private schools near the city, offered me a job. It seemed like the perfect situation. I'd be teaching Spanish. I *wouldn't* be teaching music as I had been doing for the previous three and a half years. I could no longer stand the assumptions (some implicit, some explicit) that some colleagues made about music teachers (it was all we knew how to do, our only job was to have fun all day, we couldn't be trusted in any other academic capacity, etc.). The job became stifling—never because of the students, however. I could even deal with the parental helicoptering. The children were the reason that I went to work every day. Bright souls, bright minds. Creative and curious spirits. The adults were the ones who had preconceived ideas about what a music teacher was and did; they were the ones who openly questioned my intelligence and expertise in the subject (even with degrees from Oberlin . . .).

"Well, according to the MENC (Music Educators National Conference) standards for choral spaces, the rooms need, ideally, a minimum of twenty-five square feet per student. I know that sounds like a lot, but if you consider the movement that happens in a choral classroom outside of just standing and singing, it makes complete sense," I said one day in a new facilities planning meeting. I had met with a grad-school professor of mine, and done the research. I was prepared.

"How do *you* know that?" asked Jeremy, the assistant head of the middle school.

"What do you mean? The MENC is our national music teachers' organization. How would I not know? Also, I talked to the director of the choral program at Lehman College, who, um, teaches *choral teachers* . . ." I responded with a little bit of an attitude.

"I guess we'll take that under consideration," he said, turning away and moving on to another item on the agenda. This meeting, along with other slights and judgments, was my cue. Eventually I could no longer suffer through the crushing feeling of not being considered as an equally adept and intelligent teacher. I had pictured myself continuing to build the middle-school music program for years to come, and because of this I had invested every ounce of my creative energy into it. My students made their own gourd instruments from scratch, formed blues bands, staged their own drama productions, and created wonderful music, wherever they were on the musical learning spectrum. Some of my colleagues failed to see this. It was time to move out of teaching music and find a way to engage my other passion for languages.

———

Unless you're in the actual city of Baltimore, or in one of the DC suburbs with a good public-transportation infrastructure, living successfully without owning and constantly being in a car is nearly impossible. Perhaps I was naïve about moving somewhere I had assumed would have a similar infrastructure to New York City. I had no idea that I would be leaving my wandering feet back home in New York for a few years.

Living near Baltimore alone with a small child would be difficult (Cito stayed behind in New York to continue working at a trucking company so that he would have no interruption in his employment), but I knew the move was good for my career. I had to learn how to drive, get a license, find a suitable apartment while not having a stellar credit history, and move my son and myself to a place with no family nearby. I was determined to make it work.

Before moving to Maryland, I had no driver's license to speak of, let alone a permit. I had only my state ID, because in a pedestrian-ruled city like New York, no one really *needed* to drive anywhere. I had friends who would transport me back and forth from college, and if I needed to travel somewhere, I could always hop on the Metro-North, a Greyhound bus, the New Jersey Transit, or the MTA.

So there we were in a large "luxurious" (by the rental company's standards) apartment in Owings Mills, a step up from our beautiful prewar existence in one of the most diverse and eclectic communities of the five boroughs of New York City. This apartment had two bathrooms instead of one small, awkwardly angled one, a modern kitchen (no cockroaches *or* mice!), a large master bedroom with an en suite bathroom, a smaller but still generously sized second bedroom (that

Rashid would sleep in for a grand total of maybe five days), a decent living room, and an actual dining room!

Working at the Park School would allow me to afford high-quality childcare without selling off my organs and the contents of my ovaries. Although not perfect, the new job would be a great situation for me, and eventually my little family.

Perhaps the biggest bonus of moving to Baltimore was that our almost-brand-new apartment complex had a spacious outdoor pool (that I would use regularly during the summer) and a small fitness room with an elliptical machine, a StairMaster, and a rowing machine. I wouldn't have to join a gym to continue with my fitness endeavors. Furthermore, my school also had a beautifully appointed fitness center with racks of weights, a choice of treadmills, and other cardio machines that I was free to use when I wasn't teaching.

Even with no family nearby, I learned to survive. I quickly realized that with the highest-quality childcare that I could afford (Ms. Barbara's in-home day care and school was second to none!), parenting alone would prove arduous and daunting, and at times impossible. With an as-yet-undiagnosed asthma sufferer on my hands, completing a full week of teaching was a challenge most weeks. I spent many days at home caring for a feverish, coughing, achy child who would eventually pass whatever bubonic plague he had to me. I would then contract the illness and pass it right back to him. We continued this back-and-forth sharing for the three years we spent just south of the Mason–Dixon Line.

At the Park School, the students called many of the teachers by their first names. There were meetings upon meetings about meetings. During one workshop in which we discussed the notion of rigor in learning at length, I likened the school's culture to a teaching cult.

I taught in both the middle- and lower-school divisions, some days standing in the freezing cold on playground duty and other days holding court in my middle-school classroom with hormonal and needy preteens.

"Señora: *¿Cómo se dice* 'girls are mean' *en español?*" This question and others like it were part of my day-to-day grind at Park. I enjoyed the students and the challenge of teaching in an atmosphere in which the students' interests directed their time in the classroom, with a little input from me. I learned about myself too.

Do I regret uprooting my family? Not at all. Despite the difficulties we endured as a family (in addition, Cito had a challenging time finding employment when he finally joined us a year and a half later), we persevered. Through continued multiday illnesses (on both mother's and child's parts) and a burgeoning hip pain that seemed to only show itself when I was feeling overwhelmed and stressed out, we made our lives work as best we could.

Three years later, we decided we'd had enough. I'd been offered a new position at the Purnell School, an all-girls boarding school in Central Jersey, where I'd live and work on campus.

———

Bob Carnevale was a cool dude. He had a way with words, the kind of facility and prowess that few people on this earth have naturally or can cultivate in a way that captures the spirit of humanity. He would sit at the head of the oblong table in an overly air-conditioned and dusty room at Drew University's Mead Hall and impart his wizardly wordsmithery to our class's fledgling works that yearned to be poetic.

I was excited but anxious to start a master's in Arts and Letters at the Caspersen School of Graduate Studies because it would be my first class in my second attempt at grad school (after one semester in a music education program at Lehman College, I decided that a grad-level education degree simply wasn't for me). The entirety of the summer of 2008 lay before me, and I was eager to start what would hopefully be a longer stint at the graduate level.

For that week, Bob assigned us to write a poem inspired by something mundane, à la Pablo Neruda's *Odas elementales* (*Elemental Odes*). I struggled to find something quotidian and ordinary to write about. Everything was boring and had no intrinsic meaning, I thought. But then, that's what the assignment was about, so I looked to a favorite pair of shoes for inspiration, my Dansko clogs, and immediately had a subject. I wrote the poem over the weekend and was eager to share it with my classmates:

Oda al zueco (Ode to the Clog)

> *On carpeted floors*
> *brimming with mites*
> *and smooth, dark*
> *gum amoebas,*
> *of antiseptic, miasmic halls,*
> *or sweaty hormone-laden rooms*
> *this stalwart of both*
> *stodgy and catalytic*
> *imparters of knowledge—*
> *lovers of letters—*
> *plods*
> *wordless—yet*
> *purposeful—along*
> *unfailing,*
> *hardly buckling*
> *beneath the prodigious weight*
> *of its peripatetic*
> *and magnificent burden.*

Oh shoe!

Of oiled Nubuck newness
and bovine odor,
inky black suede,
burnished brown, and
nurses' white—
a brilliant glossy patent,
a sturdy rubber sole,
and flawless instep,
bohemian step
granting external fortitude
and comfort
in your simplicity
and transparency
amid the patent disregard,
gratuitous scorn, and
smug sideways glances,
none too discreet.

Oh shoe!
Were I you.

Unfortunately, I never made it to that class on the day it was due.

"Hey, we were worried about you. You all right?" Bob asked, concerned.

"I'm fine now. I was in the ER on Monday night and didn't get back home until about six in the morning. Sorry," I said quietly to suddenly curious ears.

"What happened?" he asked.

"I thought I was having a heart attack. Obviously I didn't, but I was really scared I was going to drop dead. Sorry I missed class."

"Oh, I think I'll get over it," he said with a wry smile. "Welcome back. Glad you're okay."

———

The day before I missed class I had been driving back from my weekly gig through Lancaster County, Pennsylvania, and then through the Lehigh Valley, where I would pass signs that pointed drivers in the direction of places like Clover Hill Winery and the Rodale Institute. There were hand-painted placards on the side of the road from farm stands that read: "Shoofly Pie!" "Raisin Pie!" "Pickled Beets!" "Peaches!" "Fudge!" "Our Own Tasty Tomatoes!" "Sweet Corn!" "Watermelon!" "Sugar Peas!" The landscape varied from flat to hilly with tall white-and-red silos, field after field of corn, and side roads that led to even more expansive fields with taller silos, grazing horses and cows, houses with neatly tended gardens, and the more than occasional Amish or Mennonite family in a horse-drawn buggy.

That afternoon, I was driving with Rashid along US 222 toward Allentown, Pennsylvania, where the highway becomes a two-lane local road. A putrid chemical smell assaulted our noses as we merged onto the road and I continued driving north. A few minutes into this section of road, I began to feel a dull intermittent *something* in my chest. *Hmm,* I wondered. *What's up with my boob?* I wasn't alarmed or even concerned, although the sensation felt a tad weird and out of the blue.

A few miles later, after passing the Rodale sign, I started feeling more than something in my chest, heart side—a flash of pain and then nothing. Another flash of pain, like a cramp or spasm, like an image of cloud-to-ground lightning, quick and sharp, hitting its destination just as quickly as it relented. And then like a storm you think is over, deceptively calm, it began again, only more insistent, clamoring for attention like an only child in a room full of other children.

I drove on for a few more minutes, with the intermittent pains coming on strongly and then fading. I placed my hand over the left side of my chest, hoping the pains would subside. Thoughts rambled uncontrollably through my mind like a runaway locomotive:

Should I pull over?

Should I call 911?

Am I having a heart attack?

Is Rashid okay?

If I call 911 and they take me, what will happen to Rashid?

Why is this happening?

Why am I breathing so fast?

What is happening?

Okay, it went away, I think.

Oh no. Here we go again.

Oh my God, am I having a heart attack?

I'm having a heart attack.

I'm going to die.

I'm pulling over.

Because I can be devastatingly and annoyingly calm in emergency situations (probably learned from having to be calm, cool, and collected when surrounded by middle and high schoolers), I pulled over into a nearby parking lot and turned off the car. I took a few deep breaths to calm myself and looked back at Rashid, who was sleeping. Maybe it wasn't a heart attack. Maybe this was something different? I felt a fluttering, a quickening in the left side of my chest that was alternately light and then heavy. And painful.

Maybe it'll go away.

Maybe I won't have to call 911.

I can't take another astronomical medical bill.

I took a few more deep breaths and waited through another wave of not-as-sharp pains. After more minutes in the parking lot, I decided to continue driving home. Throughout the rest of the drive, I kept rubbing my chest on and off as if that could quell the unease and discomfort. I thought through all the signs of a heart attack that I could muster out of my frazzled and nervous brain. I tried to remember the specific signs for women because I knew they could be different. *What were they? Chest pain with arm and shoulder pain, right? Fatigue? Fast breathing? Stomach pain? Wait, no . . . burping? Dizziness?*

I don't remember the rest of the trip back home, except for periodically glancing in the rearview mirror to check in on Rashid, who had since awoken. We drove in silence. Every sensation became clearer and louder to me, and I noticed extraordinary details, almost as if the world were moving in slow motion and I was speeding through it. I identified the individual voices of NPR fame as we passed through different areas of Lehigh Valley. I heard Rashid's rapid breathing. I felt my own rapid heartbeat. Boom, boom, boom, boom, boom . . . And then a pain, more like dull discomfort, would remind me that I had something to take care of once I got home.

We arrived home at around eight at night while Cito was still at work. I immediately called my friend and colleague Kathy, knowing that her husband, William, also my colleague, would probably be able to watch Rashid while she drove me to the nearest hospital, Morristown Memorial.

"Hey, Kathy, it's Mirna," I said, trying to sound calm. But I couldn't control the slight trembling of my voice.

"Hey, what's up?" she asked, concerned. I didn't usually call my colleagues. "Everything okay?"

"Um yeah, well . . . no. I think I might be having a heart attack. Um . . ."

"Mirna!"

"Can you drive me to the hospital?" I said, beginning to cry.

After a few seconds of muffled sounds, Kathy returned. "I'll come and get you, and William will bring Rashid to our house. Are you sure you don't want to call an ambulance?" she asked in her always-sprightly tone.

"I'm sure."

———

Kathy arrived soon thereafter, and the drive to the hospital was a long twenty-two minutes in her green Dodge Caravan. People show nerves in different ways. I was calm (on the outside at least) and somewhat detached from my body as Kathy told nervous death jokes. I can't even remember what they were, but I thought it odd yet funny that she would tell those kinds of jokes while en route to the hospital. They did take my mind off my impending death, though.

After we checked in, I was quickly triaged and given a bed. After eight hours of blood tests, EKGs, blood-pressure readings, and visits from various hospital personnel, including the handsome Indian doctor on call who told me I had probably been suffering from an anxiety attack, I was discharged and sent home with my husband at about five in the morning. The ER doctor referred me to a cardiologist for follow-up. My C-reactive protein level was high, which could certainly mean a heart attack or something else in the future.

On the ride home from the hospital, Cito cradled my hand in his. He was wearing the same green Ecko Unlimited button-down shirt that he had been wearing when I had been in the emergency room for a miscarriage a few years earlier.

"You gonna be all right? You scared me. I thought my wife was dying. Man, I was so scared. Miss Kathy said you was in the emergency room. Man, I'm so happy you are okay. I was so scared. Everybody in this country work too hard, no breaks. Work, work, work. Wake up and work. Eat and work. Everybody sick, man. It's crazy."

"I think I'm okay . . ."

I fell asleep and woke up startled a few minutes later, my thoughts rambling again.

Anxiety? Me? I don't have anxiety. That shit is for people who can't handle shit. I can handle anything and everything. There's no way I had a panic attack. I don't panic about anything. And inflammation? What the fuck does that even mean? I knew what inflammation was, but I had never heard about it in this specific context via blood work. *Is this some new gimmick, the latest en vogue terminology for something commonplace? What the hell?*

"Hindsight is twenty-twenty," they say. It's true.

I realized that stress and its cousin, anxiety, were a part of my daily life.

My job at Purnell was highly stressful.

I was a dorm parent on duty many nights during the school week and on the weekends.

I taught a full schedule of Spanish classes.

I was in grad school.

I had a son who was sick all the time, so much so that we worried he would have to make up days during summer school.

I was also sick *all the time*. I had what seemed like a two-year-long sinus infection, complete with colds and flus that Rashid and I would toss back and forth to each other like passing drills in basketball.

Both Cito and I had erratic hours.

I worked every single weekend either at school or tutoring, or giving private music lessons.

I didn't sleep and neither did Rashid.

I had hip bursitis.

In the midst of doing what I loved to do and being what I thought I wanted to be—busy, outwardly calm and collected, doing everything and being everything to everyone—I had forgotten one important person: me. I hadn't noticed that in my quest to be different, in my quest to *not* be the martyr that all the women in my family seemed to be, I had quickly become just that.

———

A week later I was in Dr. David Freilich's office for another assortment of tests and questions that included a thorough EKG with wires seemingly attached to the entire surface area of my body, a battery of blood work, and what felt like five hundred forms to fill out with information detailing my health history, family health history, sleeping patterns, diet, and job.

After some nerdy banter including geographical trivia questions with an intern and me, Dr. Freilich cut to the chase.

"Well, you didn't have a heart attack," he said in a very Brooklyn sort of way, with an appropriately thick and comforting accent.

"Yeah, I know. Thank God."

"But let me ask you this." He leaned in and looked me in the eyes.

"Yeah?"

"How old is your son?"

"Five," I said.

"Do you wanna see him grow up?"

Silence. How could I answer this question without sounding like a bumbling idiot? How could I not have known that my health had been spiraling out of control, so much so that my body needed to stop me in my tracks with this urgent and painful message? How could I have missed all the signs? Debilitating hip pain, headaches, colds, viruses, an expanding waistline, an inability to sleep deeply and fully, poor dental health, and an annoying habit of saying yes to everything asked of me.

"You'll need to change your lifestyle drastically." He dragged out the word *drastically*, Brooklyn-style.

"Okay." That was all I needed to hear, someone to tell me I was doing too much, working too hard, and that I was essentially killing myself.

"Also, I'd like you to lose fifteen pounds by November."

"Done. Got it." At this point, I would have agreed to selling my left kidney if it meant I would live healthier and see my son grow and flourish. Rashid's health largely depended on my own physical and mental health. It was time to make this connection, one that I knew intellectually but had forgotten in the midst of creating a life for my family.

I walked out of the office feeling as though I had just missed the death train. I felt relieved—although the thought of having a cardiac event was scary, I could help prevent the real thing from happening with some immediate changes to my lifestyle. The danger of imminent death was clear and present. I had to change, and I had to change right then and there. I needed to make sure that I didn't die before I witnessed my son grow up and become the greatest man he could be. I knew exactly what I needed to do.

———

A few weeks later, I followed up with my primary-care physician in Pottersville, New Jersey, determined to collect all the information I could about how I was doing metabolically. The doctor performed more EKGs and blood tests, and the results were fairly similar to those that had been done both at Morristown Memorial Hospital and at the cardiologist's office: inflammation, elevated cholesterol, okay blood sugar, and normal blood pressure (surprisingly low for someone my size).

The doctor left the room to allow me to get dressed and reconfigure. As I was slipping my cold hands through the armholes in my T-shirt, I glanced over at the counter and saw what she had written in big, doctorly cursive:

MORBID OBESITY

My spirits sank.

I had never considered myself to be morbidly obese. In fact, that term hadn't even existed for me until the doctor used it to diagnose my condition. Now "morbid obesity" defined me to that doctor.

Having this diagnosis and descriptor added to my name made me cringe. I thought that people who were morbidly obese weighed like four or five hundred pounds. The condition belonged to folks with stomachs hanging past their privates, with double and triple chins jiggling as they laughed, with mobility issues that caused them to need to waddle around or ride in an electric chair at the supermarket. Of course, these are all stereotypes of people who live in big bodies, some of which do describe *some* people with morbid obesity. I suddenly found my mind wandering there. With these images in my head, I began in earnest to plan my return to fitness and overall health right then and there. Dr. Freilich had struck the proverbial match, but my primary-care doctor had put the match to the fuel and set my brain afire. I was ready to lose significant weight and make the necessary changes in other areas of my life. I was ready to start running and training again after an almost-four-year hiatus.

To start, I removed the clothes and boxes from the side bars of the treadmill that I had purchased four months previously to go with my Total Gym. I hadn't yet used either item.

Okay, I'll do a mile and see how that goes. The screen read 17:45 after I had sweated through probably the ugliest, least elegant, and most difficult mile of my life. What had happened to me? What had I done to myself? I clearly had some work to do.

I looked online and immediately found a local 5K race to train for, knowing that I would need to run regularly, and remembering that running also made me feel great. I also needed a goal to work toward so that I wouldn't be completely consumed by the intricacies of losing weight. I knew myself, and I knew how obsessive and rigid I could get. I wanted to enjoy the process and savor each victory that came along.

I started to train with a sense of urgency that I had never had before. I bought books—*The Complete Book of Running for Women* by Claire Kowalchik and *Running for Mortals* by John Bingham and Jenny Hadfield—and did run-walk intervals until I could run for thirty minutes straight. I dug out all my exercise videos—*Yoga Booty Ballet, Slim in Six, Tae Bo, Crunch* everything, *Rodney Yee Yoga*, and every *Biggest Loser* video I could get my hands on. I even scoured Netflix for anything fitness related.

My friend and colleague Nikki, who also wanted to commit to a health-and-fitness program over the summer, joined me in my insanity. We played tennis in the mornings and afternoons, we ran together—doing as many as three 5K races a week—we scouted out different local gyms, and she brought over her own videos (Denise Austin, *Hip Hop Abs*, and other Shaun T delicacies). We were serious and committed to succeeding at both weight loss and improving our health.

"So, coach, what's on the menu for today?" Nikki asked in her loud, slightly raspy voice.

"Okay, we're gonna run three miles first. Then we'll play tennis for an hour. Did you bring your racket? Oh, and afterwards we're gonna go to the gym to do some weight lifting. And then we'll take a break and eat lunch. Let's do some lesson planning in the afternoon and then finish up with a video. How about Denise Austin? Okay? Oh, and by the way, there's this 5K in Morristown tomorrow night."

Nikki sighed and rolled her eyes. "Jesus! How did I agree to this? You're killing me! I die a slow death every day. Every single day! You. Are. Nuts."

She became accustomed to my fitness antics, though. I had a written plan every day, and she made sure that we did everything on the list. One day, however, I was too tired to finish even half of what I had planned. I had gotten carried away.

"Dude, I'm done. I can't even lift my arm, it's so sore," I said, making a show of how tired I was, slumping my shoulders and sighing deeply.

"Um, as I recall," Nikki said matter-of-factly, "we finish everything on the list. Lemme see." She reached for the list, but I stuck it in my sports bra.

"You are the worst! I hate you. We have to finish!"

"For real? It's only one more set. Four is too many. Can we just stop? I'm dying."

"You are not dying. Aren't you trying to lose weight? Aren't you trying to *not* die?" Nikki had a way of reminding me of things.

"Jesus. Fine." We finished the last set and rewarded ourselves with a glass of white wine that evening.

I kept a loosely organized food journal to track the types of nutrients I was consuming, and she used an online meal service. I was conscientious about cooking my own food after having eaten all year in the school's dining hall, and made sure to burn more calories than I was consuming, even though I was fully aware that calorie consumption was only part of the picture. I knew that reclaiming my health would be a long journey and that change would come slowly. I was ready and willing to jump in headfirst.

———

Mirna Valerio

The weight loss came. By the following summer, I had lost around thirty pounds. My pants size decreased from a size 24/26 to a size 22 and then to a 20 by the end of the year. By the winter of 2011, I weighed in at 240 pounds from a high of more than 300 pounds just two years earlier.

Throughout those years of my concerted effort to lose weight and regain health, the schedule during school days was grueling. I remained focused on running and other exercise to maintain my weight and continue on the path to long-term health. I joined Life Time Athletic club in Berkeley Heights, New Jersey, at which I often arrived at five in the morning. Several times a week, I hit the treadmill for a three-mile run before joining a high-intensity interval class led by military-like comedic instructor DeWayne, who made sure that everyone felt like they belonged in the class at whatever level of fitness they enjoyed, and in whatever bodies they lived in. I went to the pool to swim laps for thirty minutes afterward, showered, ate breakfast at the club, and finally headed to work. Twice a week, I went back out again for a short run in the afternoon or did a short exercise video.

These days were invigorating, and the fatigue I felt by the end of the day was overwhelming but welcome. I had worked hard to feel like I felt, with a welcome soreness throughout my body and a new ability to sleep through most of the night—sometimes, when Rashid wasn't wandering around the apartment at three in the morning.

I upped the ante by posting about my fitness successes (and failures) on my Facebook page:

20 lbs down!

Off to the wilderness for about an hour or so . . .

1hr spinning (ouch!)+1hr CRAZY cardio/sculpting class+3miles=half dead mommy

Can someone teach me how to do breaststroke? I feel like an idiot in the pool; I probably look like a really big toad. HELP!!!

4mi+1hr hatha yoga+1hr strength training+Chipotle :)
6.5 mile total today!

Today begins 31 days of fitness!!!! Exercise every day and post what you've done!!!

Missed the police escort by about 6 people today at the Westfield Turkey Trot. It's gettin' better!

Dead last. Police escort and everything, including the guy dressed as a sock puppet who ran the last mile with me!

A little rock-climbing, stream-hopping, teeter-tottering, ankle-rolling, huffing and puffing, and copious sweating made for a lovely morning on Schooley's Mtn. When they said mountain, they meant it!

The Amish Country Bird in Hand 1/2 Marathon this morning was an absolutely gorgeous course, although it was VERY hilly. The hills felt really good—never thought I would ever say that! It was also windy and cold, which made me run most of it, I guess. Worst part: well you can guess this one, was the horse shit. Best part: all the super-cute

Amish kids handing out water. Definitely doing this one next year!

Finally finished a half in under three hours!

There are people who feel like they need to run a couple of miles before a half marathon. I am not one of those people.

DayQuil+humidity+heat+general not feeling well=a DNF. Oh well, the people organizing the run were nice folks . . . 5 miles completed.

Really like long-distance running. No marathon until 2011 though. And then in 2012 maybe an ultra. Maybe.

Cut her 5K time by another 20 seconds!!!!! WOO-HOO!!
4 miles was REALLY hard today.

Finished the Woodbridge Crossroads 5K (too tired for the 10k) in 39:10, making this a PR (personal record) and the reaching of a summer-long goal to finish a 5K in under 40 mins. ALSO, people who finish 10Ks in under 40 should be shot.

4 miles plus a very slow 5K (with little Mr. Africa) = 7.1 miles WOOOOHOOO!!! and 2 nice swag bags!!

Major, MAJOR plateau. Ugh!

Did TWO SECONDS better on today's 10-miler than on her last one. How's that for a PR?
How one can run a 10-miler in a thong is beyond me . . .

Is officially under 250. OFFICIALLY! Now for that Philly cheesesteak . . . JK!

Ran 5 miles in the morn yesterday, then cut off FIVE whole minutes from her last XC 5K last night in Morris Plains. Now off to the gym—the paunch has got to go!

Thanks to South Beach phase 2, that's five pounds gone.

Dear friends and family: As I am trying to control my weight and improve my health, I ask you kindly to refrain from sharing your sweets with me. Controlling sugar intake is a big challenge for me, so I ask for your help with this. I will accept a date for a workout, however. With love and respect, Mirna

Ich bin eine MARATHONER! TOOK ME OVER SIX HOURS BUT I FINISHED!!!

Who's ready for an 18-miler this weekend?!?

18 miles run today b*itches!

Just finished the Charm City 20 Miler. Twenty miles is LOOOOOOONG . . .

Dear [Hurricane] Irene, please time your arrival to not coincide with my half marathon on Sunday morning. The evening would be best. I appreciate your consideration.

Wow, marathon training takes over your life!

R: I want you to get fired so you don't have to work.
M: Well, what would I do all day?
R: We could go to the gym and work out . . .

I started a Facebook group with some friends I had invited to share their fitness goals and journeys. We called ourselves the TIN Soldiers 365 (the Time Is Now! 365 days a year!). We posted our workouts every day, inspired each other, shared our successes and frustrations, encouraged one another, and came up with little (or big) challenges to keep ourselves motivated. We loved our group even though many of us hadn't met each other in real life. We witnessed people attempting their first 5K races, starting up a fitness regime, running marathons, undertaking their first marathons, expanding their yoga studios, and learning and practicing new poses. There was something for everyone. I lived to post almost daily in our little forum. Posting gave me a new kind of high; this external motivating factor was the icing on the fitness cake.

This group and other groups like it kept me and other group members accountable in a supportive atmosphere and steered me closer to helping others realize their own fitness goals and dreams.

I continued to drive to Maryland on the weekends to teach and tutor, but I didn't leave until after I had finished running my weekend races and taking classes at the gym. I dedicated myself to living, and with this in mind, my days were organized around my health and wellness. I finally understood that for my son to stay healthy, I had to do the same.

8

HART STREET

On summer evenings, Hart Street in Brooklyn was abustle. For weeks before the Fourth of July there would be distant and near firecrackers, M-80s, cherry bombs, Roman candles, sparklers for the scaredy-cats, and other works we probably weren't supposed to be messing with at such a young age. We kids would be out in full force playing tag while the older teens would hang on the gritty stoops, making out and talking big-kid stuff.

Along with tag we played Mother May I, Red Light Green Light, Spin the Bottle (with empty two-liter plastic bottles we'd find in someone's garbage before the folks who went around collecting bottles to return for deposit got to them), and Hide-and-Seek (although we called it Hide-and-Go-Seek). We raced up and down the block on foot, on our bikes, and on skates. The boys played Skully right in the middle of the fucking street. Someone would spray-paint a big square whose corners were boxed off and filled with numbers. Kids would collect bottle tops and fill them with melted candle wax, and when the tops dried, the kids would lie down on the ground, face close to the actual road, and try to flick their skullies into someone else's territory. I think that's how the game went.

There were other games you played in the street like stickball and handball, which was played near the stoop and further back, sometimes even across the street.

We were outside all the time, even though many of us had started to acquire rudimentary gaming systems. I'm talking Atari 2600, ColecoVision, Sega Genesis, and the Nintendo 64. There were very strict hours for play . . . definitely not on a weekday, unless you were finished with your homework and had done all your chores after dinner. If someone was watching their show, you couldn't interrupt them, even if it was *your* day to watch TV.

"Ya wanna play tag?" asked Mel, the oldest of our cousin group.

"No, cuz last time you cheated. Let's play something else," Keisha, another cousin, said in her high-pitched voice.

"What about Red Light Green Light?" I asked.

"Okay, I'm going first!" yelled Eric, Mel's brother.

"You went first last time. It's *my* turn," said Kashene, another cousin.

We got into formation—Kashene the leader stood in front of our building's stoop—and placed ourselves at a green parking pole about fifty yards up the block.

"Red light, green light, one-two-three!" she yelled at the top of her lungs.

We ran fast toward Kashene as she rotated and made herself dizzy. She stopped and pointed to whoever was unlucky enough to be moving when she opened her eyes.

"I saw you. And yer out!"

We were expected to stay outside for hours while our parents cooked, relaxed after work, did grown-up things, gossiped among one another. There were a lot of us: me, my brother, Duke, and my sister in a stroller, Allie, whom I was in charge of; my cousins Mel, Eric, Keisha, Kashene, and Uncle Nat's five kids before they moved to a beautiful five-bedroom house in Crown Heights. There was Jennifer from down the block who would join essentially every family gathering even though she was technically a friend.

Unlike many children today, our lives were such that physical activity was built into everything we did. If we weren't outside playing, we were at school in PE class or involved in a complicated game that involved a lot of running across our concrete school yard during recess.

We came home from school exhausted. But after snacking a bit and completing our homework, we were back at it, even when it became dark in late fall. Our parents knew how important it was for us to spend time outdoors, even if it was just to sit on the stoop and sit in the sun. We enjoyed each other's company, even when we bickered (which was a lot). Hart Street was a veritable playground, where we learned how to sprint up and down the block at full speed, and where we developed lifelong friendships with all the kids who lived on the block.

Summers, our group of cousins would leave early in the morning to catch free breakfast at our zoned elementary school, P.S. 123 (because our school was in a poor neighborhood, breakfast and lunch were free even after school let out for the summer months). Being in the dark basement lunchroom felt weird with all the lunch ladies in their hairnets and white aprons smiling at us and handing out the morning food, which usually consisted of a processed egg product on dry English muffins, a piece of fruit, maybe some odd-tasting sausage for protein, and either a small red container of whole milk, a brown chocolate milk (if we asked nicely), a pink "strawberry" milk, or a blue low-fat milk. I didn't like the way milk smelled like wet dog, so I usually didn't drink it.

We sat down and quickly ate our breakfast from the yellow foam plates divided into sections—the big one for the main part of the meal and several smaller areas for foods like fruits, the occasional cookie, and so forth.

After breakfast, we went outside to Maria Hernandez Park right across the street from the school until the sun became too warm for running around. We then went home, rested a bit, finished some chores while pretending that we were having trouble making our beds (making the top bunk look neat isn't easy), and then reconvened as a cousin group, yelling "Hurry up, ya," in the hallways and up the stairs so we could make the most of lunchtime.

We'd have to travel farther for the free lunches. We'd start out at J.H.S. 162, eat quickly, and then head over to P.S. 86 a few blocks away. P.S. 274 was next, followed by J.H.S. 291. We always collected as many desserts as we could, such as little square brownies wrapped in plastic or a stack of three chocolate-chip or oatmeal-raisin cookies (we preferred the chocolate-chip over the oatmeal). No matter what dessert we gathered, I stuffed them all in the back of Allie's stroller, doling them out to everyone at various parks. Sometimes we hit more schools for lunch; other times when it was raining we'd only hit one school and head back home to annoy the adults because it was too wet to be outside and we might catch cold.

After our daily lunches, it was park time. Which one would we go to today?

Should we walk most of the way home and go to the park up the block with the track? The park around the corner or the one by Palmetto? They got sprinklers there.

No, let's go to the pool by the Marcy Projects!

No, how about the one that's real far away by all those Polish people?

Let's just go to the school yard.

No, that's boring.

We'd end up at some park, swinging, seesawing, doing flips off the monkey bars, pretending we were Nadia Comaneci. We'd slide down the "fire" poles, burning our skin on the hot metal, but then we'd do it again, thinking that somehow this time would be different. We pushed each other really high on the swings. We stood on them and pumped ourselves, secretly wishing we would somehow pump hard enough to make the swing circle the pole above our heads. Sometimes two of us would be on the same swing—one would stand and pump while another sat and pumped, extending and retracting their legs so that we could swing as high as possible.

"Push me, but don't push too hard," Keisha said as she began to pump her legs back and forth.

"Pump your legs more!" I commanded. "Higher! Go higher. Pump!"

She swung her legs, gaining enough momentum to stand up and pump her legs even more. This is where the fun began. I moved out of the way so she could soar.

"Don't pump too hard. You gonna fly off the swing!"

What we were doing was dangerous. There were few adults at the park, and we took risks for the thrill and adrenaline rush we would get from swinging at high speeds. We were free and unencumbered, moving through our lives with verve, energy, and a passion for being outside.

When we got tired, we would dig into our stash of treats from the free lunch and sit on the park benches in the shade; then we'd start all over again until our legs and arms were sore, our hands smelled like metal or rubber, and our skin was dirty, hair sweaty, and our clothing bore the marks and tears of a fine day at the park. If it was really hot out, someone would figure out a way to open the fire hydrant so that the whole block could cool off.

> *We soaked our feet*
> *in rivers at the curb*
> *clear, cool*
> *rushing over*
> *our wrinkled toes*
>
> *Cars drove by*
> *slowly for a wash*
> *the water beating*
> *on closed windows*

We filled five-cent bottles
and splashed each other

We ran, chased,
caught, hugged.
We moved.
We learned.
We grew.

9

THE GIFT OF MY MOTHER'S LEGS

Most people think of bedrock—yes, I mean geology—as an almost impenetrable, impermeable, hard, and unyielding level of ground that is pretty much indestructible. Most times it is, until groundwater seeps through cracks in what scientists call "bedding planes." It might take decades, but the area of bedrock most affected by the seeping groundwater will eventually begin to dissolve, creating fissures, cracks, and sinkholes like when the earth suddenly opens up, sucking people and parts of their homes into dirt- and rock-filled vortices. Sinkholes, for the most part, are irreparable, wreaking havoc on lives and livelihoods and devaluing homes and homesteads. They destroy foundations and other aspects of the integrity of home construction and well-being to the point that insurers are unwilling to insure properties near them.

———

My mother, Joann Taylor, has thick, stocky legs, like the gnarled trunks of centuries-old trees. She's embarrassed by her beautiful brown legs and hides them most days with long pants and capris. Being a black woman with a generous amount of culturally granted pride in being curvy, she doesn't hide their overall shape, though—this is tantamount to blasphemy. She isn't confident that most folks will appreciate the tangled webs of thick varicose veins by her knees that frame the sides of her legs. She doesn't want anyone to see the veins or the loosening skin that allows the fatty tissue to droop down and be a bit lumpy, pulled strongly by gravity and a life lived on her feet, always at the service of others.

She has always been a slow walker, but not because *she* is slow. In fact, the woman can move with a deafening speed, particularly when supervising her staff in Starbucks, setting up and taking down booths for conferences at the Jacob Javits Convention Center, catering a massive family event, or rescuing a child (mine) who decides he's going to run out into the middle of a bus-filled city street in downtown Brooklyn. She runs fast, feet moving at a blazing speed, captures said child, admonishes him, hugs him tight, nuzzles his nose, and resumes her deliberate walking down the crowded, commercial blocks of Fulton Mall.

As kids, we made fun of how slowly she and my aunt Sherry walked everywhere. An errand to the supermarket on Knickerbocker Avenue sometimes took hours. Even though Sherry lived right above us on the second floor of our apartment building, they didn't spend much time in each other's homes because they both had large families. Sherry had her own two boys in the apartment and Eric (whose father was my mother's brother, though he and Sherry weren't married), along with her sister Chinkie and Chinkie's daughter, Keisha. Even though Sherry and my mother weren't blood relatives, everything they did together suggested otherwise. They were the kind of sister duo that was inseparable, best friends.

The two would walk to Scaturro's market together, talking and laughing, most likely making fun of other people in the family or gossiping about the people up the block. My mother has a distinguishable chuckle, and Sherry had a way of summing up different situations with an accusatory, questioning, damning, or laughter-inducing *"Mmm!"* that sounded a bit like a car racing off in the distance at full throttle. We could all guess, just by the tone or gist, what was being discussed at length.

On their walks they would compare notes on the kids and other subjects in their lives: who was being bad in school, who was excelling, who was still peeing the bed, who had to stay at the table and finish their lima beans, which man had upset or abandoned them, which brother/sister/aunt/uncle was on what drug, who was pregnant again, whose asthma was still acting up, who got left back, who had a new job, who needed to learn how to cook, who was going to finish their GED first, who wanted a better life—the list was almost endless.

My mother and aunt had a relationship that was closer than that of sisterhood. My mother's brother Butchie and Sherry had Eric together. (Eric would succumb to congestive heart failure at the age of twenty-seven, another victim of poor health spurred on by family health history, poverty, lack of education, and extreme service to others at the expense of self.) To all of us, Sherry was our aunt, and all her kids were our cousins. We grew up together, celebrated birthdays in each other's apartments, and walked to and from school in a big loud, raucous group. We were family.

They would amble slowly down the block, past the rows of beige apartment buildings with wrought-iron fences on the sides of the stoops. Some buildings still had signs on them, vestiges of the 1970s that read "BOMB SHELTER" near basement entrances. One corner had a Laundromat where people dried their clothes (most people had washing machines in their apartments). After turning the corner off Hart Street and onto Knickerbocker, a person had many choices for how to spend his or her money—Tony's Pizza (still the best in Brooklyn); a Korean fruit market; various shoe stores; a fish market; Circo's Pastry Shop, whose vanilla- and anise-flavored goodies you could smell from blocks away; a Salvation Army; an Italian ice-cream shop (whose pistachio ice cream was to die for); a place that sold the best mortadella and *soppressata* this side of Brooklyn; a couple of pharmacies; a liquor store that was also a New York State Lotto hub whose owner was bitter and disgruntled; and a place where a person could buy an entire dinette set for a hundred bucks.

Every neighborhood has to have an anchor, a place where people can find community, gossip about the latest events (*Who had a heart attack? Who died? Who bought a car? Who's in jail?*), and shop daily for family provisions. Scaturro's was the place where the store manager, Dennis, would greet people. Need the best fruit? He could hook you up. Need milk that wasn't nearing expiration? He would go to the back and get it for you himself. Everyone shopped at Scaturro's. The produce was plentiful, cheap, and unbruised. They had real food, meats from local New York and New Jersey farms, and a deli that topped many of the other delis in the area. Italian women and men worked the deli, made you Italian sandwiches, and understood when you asked for just a quarter pound of ham because that's all your family could afford.

My mother and Sherry found a community there—one in which they were loved, respected, and treated like human beings (unlike when they had to visit the Public Assistance Office, for example). They could feed their children wholesome meals every single day of the week, even with public assistance. These women worked hard to make sure their kids, husbands, and boyfriends were well fed, despite the frequent dire financial circumstances they often faced.

They made sure that their families never went without food, even if it meant putting pride aside and accepting USDA canned pork, pork and beans, and whatever other surplus food they could get. When times were good and jobs were plentiful, both women worked late hours, allowing themselves a few luxuries like buying us new shoes and clothes that fit, and maybe something for themselves.

Sherry had a massive, fatal heart attack in 1993 at the age of thirty-seven, providing a shock from which almost no one in the family has recovered. She dealt with high blood pressure and other health issues for a long time and hadn't been feeling well in the months leading up to the event that would leave five children parentless. My mother, her best friend, ran upstairs when Sherry's oldest son, Mel, called for help from the top of the hallway stairs. She tried her best to revive Sherry, giving her chest compressions until the ambulance arrived. But Sherry was already dead. November 12, 1993.

Both women worked when they could find work and stayed at home when they couldn't, all the while remaining the primary caregivers in their respective families. They washed clothes, mopped floors, tended to their partners, cared for their aging parents and other infirm relatives, cooked, shopped, showed up to school events, and when they could splurge, took us all to Rockaway Beach or Coney Island. Except for the occasional gift for themselves, they rarely took a break from a busy life. They took great pains to ensure their families' comfort and success, but this came with a tremendous cost. Sherry died in service to us all. She is one of the family members whose name I invoke and whose memory I carry when I run. I run for them.

———

My mother has qualities that I have always desperately wanted to emulate, but I have failed to do so repeatedly. She is generous, kind, selfless, cheerful, positive, and faithful. She is willing to give you the *literal* clothes off her back and shoes off her feet. She will even give away her children's clothes to those who need them more. She is a consummate teacher. Every moment is a teachable moment—whenever she is around children, especially elementary-aged kids, everything is a lesson. Tripping and falling becomes a lesson in physics and a reference to Isaac Newton. Being engrossed in the game of memory becomes a language-building and word-association game. Anything and everything was fodder for Joann School. Okay, sometimes her lessons were nauseating and a little bit overkill, but she is a teacher, and a good one at that. I often find myself doing the same.

My mother loves everyone, even teenagers. She enjoys trying new foods, is adventurous, and is willing to go camping with me, her crazy daughter. She is my number-one cheerleader at races—standing for hours in the heat and humidity of some faraway forest to crew for me just because I asked, and because she wanted to experience something new, be in a place that was a far cry from Brooklyn, and meet diverse people. She listens intently, even when many people would shut others out. Perhaps most importantly to my selfish self, she is the most phenomenal cook in the family. People are drawn to her, this woman who didn't complete junior high school, this woman whose entire life comprised raising children, her own and others'.

My mother is the bedrock of our family.

As the youngest girl in her family, she frequently bore the responsibility of minding most of her older siblings' children. Considering that the oldest of the bunch, Uncle Nat, and his wife had five children, and that her other brothers and sisters each had one or two children of their own, my mother had many faces to clean and butts to wipe. She'd be in the house alone with a large or small gaggle of children with clothes to wash and sleepy eyes to put to bed.

When my mother was a young girl, her older siblings would drop off their children before going, sometimes for days at a time, to party and enjoy some time to themselves. My mother was left to fend on her own with several children of varying ages and condition of hair-done-ness. She also grappled with protecting her own mother from the ills of her worsening alcoholism and tendency to hightail it out of the house to drink and party with friends.

My mother was responsible for so many tasks and was so generous in the face of the following, much of which I categorically don't enjoy:

- Babysitting little children
- Braiding hair
- Playing games with little children and entertaining them for hours on end
- Helping people who wasted her time
- Preparing every meal for everyone in the family
- Dealing with people who actively impinge on the physical and emotional well-being of others while simultaneously being completely and utterly self-serving
- Picking other people's children up from school
- Bathing and putting little kids to bed
- Dealing with people who continue to expect you to give of yourself, especially when you have nothing left to give, and that includes *fucks*

That said, today I can't imagine having the patience and good heart to have endured the burden of a childhood lived almost entirely in the service of others. I'm amazed that my mother displays almost no bitterness, anger, or ill will toward the family members that abused her time; of course, they probably saw nothing wrong with it, robbing her of a fulfilling adolescence and young adulthood by placing her with the huge responsibility of childcare. Wrapping my head around the responsibility and day-to-day care of other people's children at the expense of my own childhood is something I can't understand. My mother made sure that her children wouldn't suffer the same fate.

In Atul Gawande's *Being Mortal*, a brilliant book on mortality and the peculiar obsession with extending lives at the expense of *quality* of life, the author's research into what allowed elderly people to continue living fulfilling (if not long), independent, autonomous lives opens up what I consider a Pandora's box of female suppression. The youngest female children were expected to assume the caretaking responsibilities of the aged. I'm angry and sad for my mother and countless other women who suffered (both knowingly and unknowingly) from a system that could only view them as baby-makers, babysitters, and caretakers of the elderly. Their worth was seen in their ability to care for other human beings.

No wonder so many women of my mother's and grandmother's generations are physically ill; these women who are the bedrock of their respective families have cracked and fissured. Their foundations crumble and they become sick from years, decades even, of standing and bending and folding and cooking and shouldering without a second thought—an automatic erasure of self, self-worth, health, and longevity, like the bedding planes eroded by seeping water.

My mother's incredible magnanimity and selflessness have manifested in her physical body. My mother is diabetic and hypertensive and has issues with mobility. Her big, beautiful brown legs that have borne the burden of many a child, adult, and elderly person are fatigued, almost as if they've had enough. Those legs bear the scars of the entire family, the burden of having been born into a poor family, the psychological weight of not having a high school diploma, and the onus of worrying about wayward members of the extended family.

Those legs also stood strong to carry her own sleeping children, holding us up, providing a firm place to rest our heads, protecting us from falling, standing at school plays and Juilliard recitals, and walking the walk of the mythical strong black woman everyone needed her to be. From those strong legs sprang children with legs that will carry an entire new generation, and I hope it's a generation that won't need to carry the weight of the next at the cost of their own health and wellness.

Joann Taylor's thick legs are the legs from which I come. I can only hope to honor the gift of her legs as I run, carrying myself, the memories of those who are gone, and the weight of the next generation for which I am responsible.

10

Heart, We Won't Forget Him

On February 22 of 2012, Nikki and I had just finished our second day of working with our students on a Habitat for Humanity house in the Ninth Ward of post-Katrina New Orleans. We were nestled in our hotel beds dozing off when my mother called to inform me that my uncle Greg had just had another heart attack.

"And this time . . . he didn't make it," she said in between deep, hoarse sobs and shudders, barely able to get out the words. No one in the family had expected this news, at least not now.

"He, he . . . he died at Brooklyn Hospital. It was another heart attack. My brother . . ." She continued to sob, the pillar of strength, the bedrock of our family. "He's gone. My little brother's gone."

After watching football at a friend's house, Greg got into the car he'd borrowed from his daughter Tina and was about to head home when he began to feel a strange sensation of suffocating pressure in his chest; he had experienced this years before during his first episode of cardiac failure. Nervous, and increasingly breathless, he called Tina on his cell phone.

"Tina, I'm getting that feeling again. I can't breathe," he said between shallow breaths.

"I'm gonna call 911. Where are you? Dad! Listen to me, okay? Stay there and don't move!" Tina commanded, her own heart beating furiously.

"There's a . . . cop on the corner," Greg gasped. An NYPD officer, whom we refer to as Officer Angel, happened to be on the beat nearby. Greg waved him over, explaining that he might be having a heart attack. The officer saw that he was in distress, summoned the EMS, and until the ambulance arrived made a valiant effort to calm and reassure Greg as his lungs filled with thick fluid and his heart struggled to keep pumping. The medics arrived and sped to Brooklyn Hospital, lights and sirens blaring, Officer Angel following closely in Tina's car. He would leave the keys with the hospital staff and disappear. Greg died almost immediately after arriving at the hospital, at the age of fifty-three. His heart had had enough.

Uncle Greg's death was shocking, and even years later, reliving the middle-of-the-night phone call and my mother's heartbreak still hurts. Speaking now with his daughter Tina and son DJ and wondering why a soul as gentle and family-bound as his is no longer with us continues to be difficult to grasp.

Some deaths are expected while others happen unexpectedly—and you mourn. Somehow you outgrow your grief and continue to remember the belated fondly, pausing every now and then to smile privately at some memory. Uncle Greg's death was different; it was as if we had all suffered the suffocation of congestive heart failure. We had all felt the earthquake of his passing, his sudden departure. It left a profound, unhealable wound in our family's heart, a black hole that sucked the life out of every family gathering as we grappled with the absence of this vital life force, this funny and complicated human being who, even if you were one of the black sheep in the family, made you feel comfortable, loved even.

———

In May of 2005, a few years before Uncle Greg's death, I was driving my old black '96 Pontiac Grand Am (on whose sides the previous owner had painted thin red-and-white racing stripes) down to Maryland after spending the weekend in Brooklyn. In addition to Rashid, who was about to turn two, my fourteen-year-old brother, AJ, was also traveling in the car. He often came and hung out with us to enjoy some time away from Brooklyn. On this trip, however, I helped him memorize Langston Hughes's "A Dream Deferred," write a poetic analysis, and write/practice an oral presentation on the life and work of the Harlem Renaissance pioneer.

Just as we were about to enter the part of the New Jersey Turnpike where the exits seem like a hundred miles apart, Jenny, the Pontiac, decided to have a temper tantrum. She started spewing a thick, sweet-smelling white smoke into the car and leaking a stream of orange-colored fluid onto the roadway. I immediately pulled over, not even checking my mirrors or blind spots, and shut the car off. Jenny was about to explode, I thought.

"AJ, get out!" I yelled. He unsnapped his seat belt and stumbled out of the car, nervous.

I jumped out of the driver's seat and went around to the back door to unbuckle Rashid from his car seat. My hands shook violently.

"Mirna, hurry up. It's leaking!"

"I'm trying!" I finally managed to pick Rashid up and pull him out of the car. He started to scream. We collected ourselves on the shoulder of the highway and tried valiantly to calm down. The smoke began to dissipate in the car, but an orange substance leaked profusely from Jenny's undercarriage.

"So what we gonna do?" asked AJ, his fear and uncertainty unmasked.

"I don't know." After a few minutes of cradling Rashid in my arms at the side of the road and checking in on AJ, I had the presence of mind to call my insurance company. The woman I spoke to talked me through what I needed to do.

"First of all, are you safe?"

"Yes. Um, for now. We're on the shoulder of the Jersey Turnpike," I answered. We were safe. The car hadn't actually blown up.

"Okay, we can't send anyone out because you're on the interstate. Here's what you'll need to do. Call 911 and tell them your car broke down on the highway, and they'll take care of it."

I followed her directions and, a few minutes later, a state trooper stopped by to ask if we were doing okay and to let us know that a tow truck was on the way. We stood outside, and the air became cold. A couple in a dark-gray minivan pulled over and asked if we needed anything. They had water, juice, and snacks if we needed them. We accepted their offering and they drove off, wishing us well.

Finally the tow truck arrived. The driver looked under the car and could tell immediately what was wrong.

"You have a coolant leak. Probably a blown gasket," he said. "That's gonna be expensive."

"Great. So where do we go? Do you take us home, or . . ."

"I take you to my garage and then you figure out what to do from there," he replied.

"Um, okay." I was grateful to get off the shoulder. It was cold, and all three of us were wearing thin jackets.

After we arrived at the garage and paid for the tow, I worked on figuring out how to get back to Brooklyn from the remote exit off the New Jersey Turnpike on a Sunday with a cell phone that was rapidly losing battery life. In a serendipitous twist of fate, that very day, Cito had started a brand-new job at a towing company. I could have waited for the truck that my insurance company would send, costing me even more money that I didn't have, or I could call Cito.

"Hey, honey. Um, we broke down on the Turnpike," I told him.

"Oh shit. Are you guys okay? Is Rashid okay? What happened? AJ, he's there too?"

"Yeah, we're okay. The tow-truck guy said something about the gasket."

In a desperate move, I asked Cito to come and pick us up, knowing that he would likely get fired for going off route on his first day at work, but there was not much else we could do.

"I know you just started your job today, but can you come pick us up? These people are closing in two hours, and then we'll have to leave. Please?"

"Aw, honey, I don't know. It's my new job. I don't know . . ."

"Can you just ask, please? We're stuck. And I don't have another hundred dollars to get back to the Bronx. Please ask."

His new boss understood, especially when Cito mentioned that his two-year-old son was also stranded. Almost three hours later, he arrived in a rickety tow truck, hitched the rapidly deteriorating Pontiac Grand Am onto the flatbed, and brought us to the dispatch station in the Bronx. His boss then drove us home.

We arrived at two in the morning to the apartment in the Bronx that we had left many hours before and fell asleep quickly on our metal-frame IKEA bed. AJ slept on our old Jennifer Convertibles pullout sofa bed that had by then started hosting a family of prewar-building-standard-issue mice. Rashid slept between Cito and me like a bridge, his head on Cito's long back and his feet on the side of my neck.

As we lay in this formation, exhausted from the vehicular excitement of the previous hours but delighted in the serendipity—the luck of it all—my cell phone rang. My phone had less than 10 percent of its battery life remaining because I hadn't yet been aware of car chargers.

I knew it was my mom. Who else would call me in the middle of the night? Someone must be dead or in the hospital, I thought. Who would it be this time? The call was staticky, but my mother's fear and sadness came through quite clear.

"Mommy? Hello? What's wrong? You okay?" I asked, preparing myself for news of some close family member's death.

"Uncle Greg had a heart attack last night," she said, her voice barely audible.

"Oh my God . . . Is he . . . ?" I expected the worst.

"He's in the PICU at Brookdale. They stabilized him," she said, both relieved and worried.

"The PICU? Like the one for kids?" I asked, my voice gravelly from the previous day's events.

"Yeah, they didn't have room for him on the adult side," she said.

"Oh my God. Okay. Um, what time do you want me to come to the hospital?" By this time, Cito had woken up and was listening to my conversation. He started rubbing my back to comfort me.

I sighed. "Okay, I'll meet you at the hospital at like ten. Call me if anything changes, Mom." I ended the call.

"What happened?" Cito asked.

"Uncle Greg had a heart attack. He's in the hospital—in the ICU."

"Oh shit. Uncle Greg? He's so young to have a heart attack," he said, shaking his head.

My job then crossed my mind. Some people in the school administration at Park had already accused me of skipping town and hanging out in New York when I was supposed to be working, so I tried diligently to do the following:

1. Not ever get sick on a Thursday, Friday, Saturday, Sunday, or Monday.
2. Not pass my cooties to my son who would then inevitably have to stay home from day care and dutifully pass them back to me.
3. Not have any family emergencies ever, especially any time during the week.
4. Not do anything that would make them think I had a life and family outside of work.
5. Just go to work sick and deal with it later (always with severe physical and emotional consequences).

There was no question in my mind that I would spend as much time at home in New York as I needed before heading back to Maryland. Family came first, and if those folks wanted to fire me because one of my favorite uncles had suffered a heart attack, then so be it. I also hadn't signed my contract for the upcoming year anyway, so really, I didn't give a crap. Again, family came first, and if they wanted to think that I was deliberately missing work because of the stress-related illnesses they had caused, then so be it.

We slept for another few hours and were relieved that there was no news. This was a good sign. We got dressed, bought buttered rolls and coffee—light with two sugars—from the grocery store on the corner, and headed down to Brooklyn to meet my mother and other family members as they swooped in from all over Brooklyn to visit Uncle Greg.

Greg had a stressful job as a maintenance worker with the New York City Housing Authority, or "the projects" as they're so lovingly called. Because of budget constraints, the NYCHA had a tendency to assign one, maybe two, workers to each building, some of them housing hundreds and hundreds of residents who, as is typical in a large city or anywhere where people actually live, generated a lot of garbage and spills. The issues he had to deal with at work—stairwells with shit and urine; broken windows; smelly, sticky-walled elevators with indefinable stains; broken locks; and stuck doors—were never ending. Each day Greg had to load multiple floors of garbage into containers, lift heavy bags onto a rolling cart, push the cart to the garbage area, and repeat the process in reverse. He also had to mop floors with caustic, industrial-strength chemicals, perform small repairs in various apartments, and maintain the outdoor areas.

He had no high school diploma, so he made up for his lack of education by toiling away at the job he'd held for almost thirty years to support his family and becoming a role model for hard work and diligence, even in the direst of financial circumstances.

Greg had a joke for everyone and every situation, even during serious occasions like funerals. He also offered heaps of praise for those in the family who were making moves, trying to do something with their lives.

"Mirna, you know we proud of you, right? You doing the thang, singing opera, teaching the kids. Yeah. You got it going on . . . Bonita Applebum . . ." This reference to the song by the rap group A Tribe Called Quest would elicit peals of laughter and waves of pride from whoever happened to be standing around.

His presence—he was slightly shorter than the average male, almost completely bald, and big-stomached—was comforting. His warm smile, much like my mother's, and aura were inviting—he lived to laugh, to dance, to eat, to share gossip, to imitate people in the family with unusual idiosyncrasies, to get people to sign this and that petition for whatever cause the local government (many of his friends were local politicians who represented various neighborhoods) was trying to gain traction for, to reminisce about the old days on Hopkinson Avenue and Woodbine Street, or to crack jokes about you right to your face.

We arrived at Brookdale Hospital and watched Greg continue to crack jokes even as he was hooked up to beeping machines, clearly experiencing pain and discomfort. He had something to say about being in the PICU, and what the hell was I wearing?

"Ain't you supposed to be home in Maryland? I thought you left," he said, suddenly wincing in pain. "And where's your coat? It's cold as hell outside."

"Don't worry about me, Uncle Greg. You're the one you should be worried about. They treating you okay?"

"Yo, this food is nasty. How they expect people to live? I'm hungry. I could use me some of your mother's yellow rice and beans, though. That rice is off the chain. When you going home?"

"Later on. We're taking the Greyhound."

"The bus? Oh no. I should get my butt right up and drive ya home."

"Um, Uncle Greg," I said, cocking my head and dramatically rolling my eyes. "You better stay here and get better, talking 'bout you gonna drive somebody home. Please. What did they say was wrong?" I asked, becoming serious.

"Doctor told me that I'm gonna need a triple bypass," he said. Later, we would find out that his heart had only been functioning at 23 percent of its capacity.

After being released from the hospital, Greg wouldn't be able to return to work, although he tried valiantly until his friend and supervisor, Patrick, drew the line. Greg was clearly sick and unable to do his job, and Patrick was worried about his friend who had worked with him for decades. Greg's heart condition pushed him into early retirement, where he became bored and restless, and he eventually signed up to volunteer with a longtime friend. Nate was a local politician with whom Greg had worked on various campaigns from time to time in the past. Volunteering would be his grand opportunity to reconnect with the working world, to do something useful and fulfilling, and to have an actual schedule—something that helped him quell his need for movement, offering interactions with humans and fulfilling the need to be needed.

He took the job as a volunteer seriously, canvassing Williamsburg, Brooklyn, for this cause and that, organizing community events, and rallying people to be more active in their particular housing developments. He was the go-to guy who knew and loved everyone, and all whose lives he touched reciprocated his affection and enthusiasm.

So it came as a terrible shock when I received that phone call in New Orleans. After hanging up, I lay in bed sobbing, causing the pillow to become drenched and cold.

"Should I call anyone at school?" Nikki asked. "Maybe someone can come and replace you."

"No," I said. I agreed to stay because we both were responsible for fifteen girls on that trip, and I felt like I couldn't and shouldn't leave them with only one chaperone for the remainder of the two-week community-service trip. "Greg will understand, I just know it."

I cried myself to sleep, my body quivering from time to time with after-sob shudders. When I woke up the next morning, my grief gained new energy. I began to cry again. I tried to busy myself with calling people in the family, but reaching anyone would prove impossible, as they were all busy notifying other friends and family about Greg's sudden death.

I ultimately decided not to attend the funeral. Trying to find a replacement chaperone would have been futile, and I also felt like I could honor Greg's memory in a different way. I went to the hotel gym that morning and worked out extra hard in his memory, pushing my own heart to its capacity and thanking it for continuing to beat, for keeping me alive, and for reminding me of that moment a few years earlier when I learned I had to change. My uncle Greg hadn't heeded the first warning—perhaps because he couldn't imagine not working, he didn't know how, he hadn't felt empowered to take care of himself, or he had been more concerned about the needs of others.

I chanted his name several times amid free-flowing tears in the empty fitness center. That day I worked strenuously on our Habitat house, and a few days later while my family and friends gathered for his funeral, I sat outside the house, out of Nikki's and my students' earshot, and wept quietly under the hot Louisiana sun.

11

Granada, 2002

Normally, walking to the foot of the Albaicín neighborhood, up the long concrete-tiled blocks of modern Granada along the Carretera de la Sierra and northwest to the old Arab section took me thirty minutes. The Albaicín is named for what used to be the Arab quarter, beneath the stunning and majestic Alhambra, the ancient Moorish fortress filled with exquisite tile work and intricate calligraphy, sublime gardens, and wide-open sunlit rooms, some with still pools, others with fountains. This palace stands towering in its enormity over the Albaicín, which seems to remain much like it may have been during the Nasrid dynasty. The neighborhood is very hilly, as the name Albaicín indicates in the original Arabic (meaning "quarter of the falconers"), much of it still paved with cobblestones. The streets have narrow houses or *cármenes* with whitewashed walls guarding cool interior patios, and upper-middle-class families who moved in after the Arabs were slowly displaced during the Reconquista.

Every weekday I made this trip, sometimes twice (if I forgot my cell phone or money—I quickly learned not to forget anything). The mornings were filled with walking the pre-sun-warmed streets of Granada, while street sweepers swept, shop owners arranged merchandise in windows (*"ORO!" "CARTERAS!" "REBAJAS!" "VENTA!"*), and bars filled with people who had stopped in on their way to work in banks, offices, stores, language schools, monuments, and tourist traps. *Café con leche, café con hielo, y pan con mermelada.*

"Gracias. 'Sta luego," they would mumble in their thick Andalusian accents as dry as the air during the hottest part of siesta.

The pavement was newly wet, and the slightly rancid smell of soaked cement that signified early morning permeated the arid air. I walked these sidewalks every day, and then up the serpentine streets (some with sidewalks, others with suggestions of them) to the language school where I would take roll, attend to any issue the students had with their homestay families or teachers, check in with the instructors, and then head off to a local restaurant to have my own breakfast of *pan con mermelada o mantequilla, un café con leche, y zumo de piña* (toast with marmalade or butter, a coffee with milk, and pineapple juice).

I dawdled for a bit to make sure there were no emergencies, hung out with my co-leader Jaime, talked politics and books, worked on planning cultural excursions to flamenco clubs or *teterías* (tearooms) to sample fruity black teas and walnut-and-honey-filled delicacies. Sometimes our trips took us to the newest *tapería* (tapas hangout) to sample traditional tapas, and *vino tinto* (red wine) for the adults. We devised walking tours of the city for the students, and we made them develop their own with a scavenger hunt so that they could practice their Andalusian Spanish, their *castellano andaluz.*

That summer of 2002 was an active one. I was determined to keep up a fitness regimen while on vacation from my real job teaching music at the Masters School. I worked as a group leader for the Experiment in International Living program, in which American students traveled to different countries for periods of up to five weeks, absorbing the language and culture from living with local families in bustling cities.

In addition to my daily walks to and from school, I made it a priority to walk to each student's homestay to meet the families. Some of the kids lived on the outskirts of the city, far from where I lived. Each family insisted that I come over for lunch so that we could have some wine with our conversation. They would learn about me, and I would learn about them and their interactions with my students over two to three hours of dining on salads filled with tuna and white asparagus generously coated with the greenest, most fragrant olive oil and crunchy sea salt. There would be bread, purchased from a local *panadería* (bakery). There was always some kind of heavier dish in the middle of the table, like a *carne asada* (roast beef), *potaje de garbanzos* (chickpea stew), or *lentejas* (lentil stew). And there was wine. For lunch. Always some table wine from a box that I swore was reminiscent of the more expensive wines that I could purchase stateside. If the host family served dessert, it would be some *natillas* (custard) or *fruta* like watermelon, grapes, plums from an uncle's plum tree *en el campo* (in the country). And then, of course, more wine.

"How is Michael doing? Is he adjusting?" I asked, ready to scribble my notes in a combination of Spanish and English in my European-style notebook.

"Well, no," Señora Ortiz Villega said. *"Es muy . . . eh . . . Americano."* (He's very, um, American.) "He won't eat."

"What do you mean? *¿No tiene hambre?"* (Is he not hungry?)

"It's too bad. He doesn't even eat *albóndigas* (meatballs)! We thought Americans loved *albóndigas!"*

"Perhaps you can ask him what he would like. I know he should eat whatever you offer, but our students are probably used to having more choices. If you offer him something he's familiar with first, I'm sure he'll eat. And then you can introduce *comida típica.* He'll come around. *Se lo prometo.* I promise."

By the time the checking in/liaising was finished, it would be around four in the afternoon and, according to the indignant expressions on the host family's faces, entirely too hot to walk back to my own host-mother's home.

"Mirna, *qué calór* (it's so hot)! You'll take a nap here. Do you want the TV? More water? A blanket? *Acuéstate*, Mirna (lie down)—you can't walk in this heat, *vale* (okay)? Your mom will understand. It's too hot. Sleep here. Here, you're family, *vale*, Mirna?" My host-mom *would* understand. That, I was sure of. She often forbade me from going out during lunch. I would then sneak out the door, tiptoeing across the cold tile floor and opening the door to a blast of Andalusian heat.

Señora Ortiz Villega lured me into a cool room with the shades closed and thin white *cortinas* (curtains) drawn so that I could enjoy my siesta in peace. I dreamed crazy dreams in a thick Castilian Spanish, imagining I was in one of the tombs at the Catedral de Granada, or hanging out in one of the caves in the small town of Guadix, stomping my feet on a wooden floor, dancing flamenco with gypsies from the Alhambra in Sacromonte. In the midst of deeply contented and red-wine-influenced sleep, the aroma of strong *café* worked slowly to disintegrate the flimsy and disconnected narrative of my bilingual dreams.

———

I ate a lot in Spain. And when I say *a lot*, I mean heaping bowls of *cocido* (a thick bean soup similar to a French cassoulet), *macarrones con salsa* (macaroni and sauce), plates of Manchego and drunken goat cheese, *albóndigas* with ground Marcona almonds, *dulces árabes* (Arab sweet treats), and fresh bread drizzled with a fruity, dark-green cold-pressed olive oil—so much oil, in fact, that I started sweating it. People were always feeding me, wherever I went.

"You're big; you need to eat."

"You're always working; you need to eat."

"You walk so much; you need to eat."

"What do you mean dinner is too late? *Para nosotros*, eleven at night is normal. Eat a few *boquerones con ajo y perejil* (fresh anchovies in garlic and parsley) and some Manchego, just before you go to bed."

"How about *un bocadillo de tortilla de patatas poco hecha* (a sandwich of potato and egg omelet, eggs a bit runny)? You'll have a long day tomorrow. I think you'll need two, *por si acaso* (just in case), *vale*, Mirna?"

I never gained weight in Spain or any other time I visited Europe. The food was fucking fantastic. There were exactly two times that I indulged in fast food—both times were at Burger King. The first time was in Córdoba, during my first trip to Spain in 1994 while on my semester abroad. The menu offered real beef burgers, some with mayonnaise and tuna . . . *tuna*? And real cheese. The burgers were huge and heavy, and they tasted, well, different. The fries were also different—thicker, less processed, and filling. In England, the second time ever I had fast food in Europe, I had a similar experience. The cheese was Emmental, not the overly processed version of what passes for cheese in fast food of the United States, but real cheese. The burger tasted like actual meat, and it probably was. Again, the fries didn't taste as if they had been dipped into a vat of preservative before they had been fried.

In Spain, the cuisine and culture was such that I had to taste everything, and for the most part, I did. I enjoy food. I looked forward to long drawn-out lunches with bottomless bottles or boxes of wine, followed by the sleepiest and most luxurious sleep, and then being awakened by coffee and reentering the awake world with *galletas* (tea/coffee biscuits) or buttery, citrus-scented madeleines.

———

After enjoying my siesta, I would get myself ready for many more hours of traipsing about the city, entertaining students, climbing the long hill to the Alhambra, rediscovering the gardens of the Generalife, and admiring and breathing in the essence of what it was to be in Spain, speaking Spanish. I lived it up: I walked, I ate. I allowed my dark skin to bake further in the hot sun. I felt so alive, energized by the sun from which many people hid, inspired by how the orange ceramic tile that covered whitewashed houses in the Albaicín glowed. I admired the majestic, outward austerity of the Alhambra, and even the newer developments of Spanish-style ticky-tacky houses, with their orange and almond trees, beautiful blue-and-white-tile details, and peaceful, shaded patios decorated with hanging flower baskets and window boxes exploding with colorful and delicate flowers.

At the end of our homestay, our in-country Spanish leaders gave our students a choice of a short weekend hike with some camping in the Alpujarras (the foothills of the Sierra Nevada), or a longer hike with much more elevation to an *albergue* just beneath the highest peak in Spain, Mulhacén, and then to summit the peak. I love to prove to myself that I can do difficult things if I can just imagine their completion; if I can envision success and do the necessary work, then I can achieve it. For the most part, this method works for me. So I chose the more difficult hike, knowing that my body would be greatly challenged. I also knew there'd be a reward of viewing up close what I could see in the distance from the hot room on the top floor of my host-mother Josefina's three-story house. In late July the mountains were still covered in snow at the very top, hence the name Sierra Nevada.

One of the teachers at the language school was an in-your-face, warm, talkative, and very expressive Spaniard with French parents. Odette was an outdoor enthusiast, and we immediately became friends, though with my introverted ways it was difficult for me to handle too much of her at one time. But her enthusiasm and generosity of spirit won me over, or perhaps it was her short, dyed red hair. *A rebel,* I thought.

"Mirna, I've heard you like the outdoors, that you're always walking through the Albaicín during siesta . . . to, eh, exercise."

"*Sí,* I love the heat, and I love the hills and the view of the Alhambra. If I could look at it all day, I would."

"It's a sight, isn't it? But every day you walk there? You're *un poco loca.*"

"*¿Estoy gorda, no?* I *have* to exercise. Also, I love it."

"Mirna, you are *perfecta* the way you are. Come with us to Monachil? The hike is difficult, but I think you'll like it."

To prepare for both the shorter and extended hiking trips, Odette planned two excursions to the Cahorros de Monachil, where we would hike along the Monachil River, across narrow, rickety footbridges among cliffs and lush greenery.

We took a series of public buses to the village of Monachil, and from the last bus stop walked up a windy road until we reached the trailhead. There were seven of us on this trip—five students, Odette, and me. Thin with a muscular and outdoorsy build, Odette walked quickly and easily up the hill, and I was determined not to lag too far behind, lest the others on the hike think that I wouldn't be able to complete it. I desperately wanted to finish it. I knew that one of the rewards in doing this hike would be adding another sensory layer to my trip in Spain, beyond the small world that my students inhabited. It would give me an alternate experience, a solid geographical understanding of where I was, and why and how things were the way they were in Spain.

I struggled a bit to keep up, but I managed never to lose sight of the rest of the group. There were no blazes on the trail that I could see, and the students were all sprightly young lads who bounced and skipped along the way up all those hills. (Who knew I'd be running this kind of terrain regularly a few years later, and that I would up the ante and run and hike up and down difficult trails for hours at a time?) To add to what I perceived as a difficult walk in the woods, we were hiking during the hottest part of the day, normally when I would be on my daily sojourn up the steep hills of the Albaicín to sit in the sun and view the old Moorish fortress. Luckily, much of the trail was shaded. The river glistened and its banks became narrower, boulders protruded more often from underneath the water, causing little eddies and mini-hydraulics beneath the increasingly rapid waters.

It felt like we were somehow in the heart of the Adirondacks, especially when the tree canopy was thick and the sun had trouble making its way through the somewhat impenetrable cover of leaves. It would be cool and misty at points and then blazingly hot where there were patches in the canopy. We stopped near a deep, clear, and cold pool to have a lunch of *bocadillos de jamón serrano, queso, tomate, y aceite, y yogur, fruta,* and tall bottles of our favorite mountain spring water from the town of Lanjarón that we had purchased at the local supermarket before heading out on our journey.

After enjoying our sumptuous long feast while sitting on warm boulders by the river, which was at this point a large, somewhat noisy stream, we took turns soaking in the natural plunge pool lined with smoothed flat stones at the bottom. The water reached up to my chest and I dunked myself repeatedly, drinking in the refreshing and curative powers of frigid mountain water after a long, dusty, sweaty, quad-crushing hike.

"I wish I could stay in Spain forever," said Michael after he had polished off two *bocadillos* with ham and thick slices of Manchego that had been marinated in olive oil. "My host-mom said I can stay with her whenever I come back to visit. I love that family," he said as he sat on a boulder, kicking water with his feet.

After resting, eating more, shooting the shit, and splashing water on each other (along with screams and peals of adult and adolescent laughter), we headed back down the trail, this time skipping and playing with each other, joking around about this or that in a combination of Spanish and English, with Odette speaking to her children (she had brought them along) in British-accented English, French, and Spanish. We reached the trailhead, proceeded down the steep road to our bus stop, and waited for our bus, tired and content.

12

MAKING PEACE WITH THUNDER

As much as I live for traipsing about in the backcountry, and even encountering bears and other notable wildlife, there are a few times when I don't feel comfortable in the forest, particularly when I'm alone and not participating in an event. In theory, I'd prefer to be nestled deeply among the trees, but in reality I always have a nagging inkling of fear and find that I can't let myself go completely. When I'm by myself, surrounded by dense, quiet flora and skittering fauna, my deeply hidden fears begin their slow ascent out of my subconscious to the *right here and now* of my mind. Every single stupid thing that I'm afraid of shows its ugly, pockmarked, snot-and-acne-covered face to me, causing me to lose focus, trip, face-plant, and look like some wild headless animal, disorienting me like those people you see running in horror movies as everything blurs.

Maybe I need those fears. I'm generally an all-over-the-place frenetic and unfocused type with all parts of me extended and dipped in different projects, disciplines, and just about anything. I become hyperfocused, sensing anything and everything around me, every leaf, every raindrop. The adrenaline that courses through my body propels me forward and helps me to keep my eyes and heart on the prize, eliminating everything else.

Fear can be crippling or it can be motivating and somewhat liberating. I choose to let it motivate me. Here is a partial list of some of my fears, some crippling and some stupid:

- Pushing the wrong button on an elevator and the doors opening to a musty, dark, and abandoned basement
- Happening upon my doppelgänger
- Running into a wild boar on a trail—bears? Been there, done that. Boars? Haven't you seen those shows on the Discovery Channel?
- Deep, murky lakes—although I will swim out in one
- The feral cats that we used to taunt and throw things at back in Bushwick hunting me down and retaliating
- A house fire in the middle of the night
- Ouija boards
- Centipedes but not millipedes
- People who believe they are mind readers and clairvoyants
- Dying in a horrific car accident and leaving my boy without a mom
- Having to work in corporate America again
- Getting stuck in a kayak—this almost happened once in Spain on a lake in the middle of nowhere
- Being stalked, robbed, and killed by a crackhead or meth head
- Diving off a pier, dock, diving board into water—clear or murky
- Getting lost on a trail at night with no headlamp and no moon
- Thunderstorms

Take thunderstorms as an example. Thunderstorms were scary to me as a child and remain scary to me as an adult. And no, I don't want any therapy. I'm perfectly happy to live in constant fear of the rumbling light show in the sky. As a matter of fact, I *love* the song "Thunderbuddies" from Seth MacFarlane's extraordinarily inappropriate-for-children film *Ted*. It exemplifies everything I've ever felt and currently feel and experience during a thunderstorm. This profound fear follows me even today (although I can hide it fairly well around people who don't know me well enough to see how my entire demeanor changes when a storm happens: listen to the odd shake in my voice and feel my skin turning clammy, the almost imperceptible tremble in my arms).

On Hart Street, my brother Duke (his first name is Ellington) and I slept on a creaky set of bunk beds, he on the bottom, and I on the top, located in what was supposed to have been the living room of our railroad apartment in Brooklyn's Bushwick neighborhood. Duke slept with the family Bible under his pillow for comfort. I slept under many blankets—an odd assortment of bleached white hospital blankets and sheets, a Strawberry Shortcake comforter, and some pseudo-wool blankets that would start pilling the instant they were removed from the package—no matter what the season was or what the temperature was in the apartment. I was always ready for a thunderstorm to suddenly erupt in late spring, summer, and early fall.

I would hide under the covers with my fingers digging into my ears, sweating profusely and unable to breathe. I would lie there, motionless, until I was so asphyxiated that I would fall asleep, but not until those last few rumbles of thunder had sounded.

Stories and explanations like the angels are bowling and God was screaming at us and crying rain-tears didn't help. They only made me fiercely and irrationally angry. Being the wannabe-precocious child that I was, I knew there were different types of weather systems, isobars, pressure systems, and clouds. I watched the news with my grandma every night at six on channel 2, so I wasn't fooled. (I was also the person who debated Bible verses in Sunday school and constantly corrected people's pronunciation, so go figure.) I'd get mad when people tried to explain the loud sounds of nature in some crazy, nonsensical manner to comfort little children. I called bullshit early on.

In the summers and late spring, I slept with a perpetual fear of being woken up during a thunderstorm. Even to this day, sometimes hours before a storm presents itself in the form of distant rumbles and any periodic brightening of the sky, I'm awake. I'm not sure what causes me to wake: the drop in air pressure or the sudden, disturbing but energetic quiet, the quieting of birds and the blanketing of all sound with heavy cumulonimbus clouds. I wake suddenly, surrounded by deep quiet, but with an insect- and birdlike instinct and compulsion to hide in my nest until the storm has passed.

———

Duke and I had been dragged to a family affair in the Cumberland houses, a public housing unit in the Fort Greene section of Brooklyn. A long barbecue had started in the morning, complete with typical Taylor family cookout fare: grilled handmade burgers; kosher beef franks; soul-food-style potato salad; macaroni and tuna salad; ribs that had been marinated overnight, grilled and basted with cheap white wine, and then slathered with doctored-up barbecue sauce; crabs steamed in beer (Colt 45 was a favorite, and one of the children had probably been sent to the corner store to pick it up—no problem in those days) and red-hot pepper flakes; chips and dip; a wilting green salad for those who were watching their weight (which was hardly ever anyone); coco rice and peas; jerk chicken; and curry goat (from the Jamaicans in the family).

The children ran around the park, playing tag, Mother May I, and Red Light Green Light in the "courtyard" at the Cumberland houses until the sky suddenly became dark and heavy with clouds. We didn't have cell phones or AccuWeather forecasts back then, so no one was prepared for the abrupt onslaught of heavy rain. The grown-ups ushered us onto the elevators that took us up to the thirteenth floor. We hurried into my aunt and uncle's apartment, in which they somehow housed five children, took off our wet tops, and waited out the storm.

Duke and I decided to look out the window from which we could see the edges of the Brooklyn Navy Yard and the East River. The thunder was still rumbling and amping up in intensity until the brightest light I had ever seen shone right in front of us. It was a ball of energy from which long isosceles triangles emanated at the sides, creating a thin flashing diamond with the dark sky as a backdrop.

And then *pow/boom/rumble/crash/stomp/kerplunk!*

The sound of the thunder was so loud that it shook us *and* the solidly constructed government-issue building. My teenaged cousin Annette stood behind us, and the jokester that she was, pushed me solidly against the safety bars on the window, as if she were trying to push me out. She snickered and I quivered, her cold wet hands against my back.

To help ease my mind, I had the wherewithal to learn about the different clouds, their formations, and what each meant. Stratus? Just rain. Nimbostratus? A persistent rain, possibly all day into tomorrow. Cirrus? My favorite. Wispy, ethereal, and cold. Way up in the sky, filled with ice crystals.

Cumulonimbus? Not my favorite. These ominous and menacing clouds, heavy with moisture, electricity, and darkness were the clouds I learned to identify first. These clouds were like an impatient and loud party with those scary high school students who smoked and made sometimes-questionable decisions, while you and your quiet, introverted self preferred to be working on homework.

The combination of sound, light, and the thought of hurling down thirteen stories created (in my adult-onset hindsight) a deep and unreasonable fear of thunderstorms that I still live with today.

———

In boarding school and college, all my close friends knew about my astraphobia. No matter what time of night or early predawn morning, I would burst out of my room and plunk myself, comforter and all, onto their dirty carpets and sleep there, soothed by the simple presence of another human being, even if I had made them angry by waking them up at some god-awful hour. Other times I called over to a friend and asked her to come to my room because I was so afraid to move from my bed. What was my fear? That the thunder gods would capture me and take me away? That the lightning would strike through the closed windows and wrap me in its frizzy tentacles and suffocate me, like a boa constrictor?

My friend would march over, reluctantly, and pull me from my bed and drag me to her room, where I would ask politely but insistently if she had an extra blanket. *Jesus, Mirna!* Sometimes I just cowered under the covers in my bed, alone, even though I had two other roommates. I still felt lonely and scared.

———

Thunderstorms often paralyze me. On a sticky, humid day in late May of 2002 as I was preparing for the next day's classes in my office at the Masters School, a storm rolled in. As I am quite the morning and evening news junkie, I should have been prepared for the evening's fierce storm. Had I paid attention to the day's forecast, I would have high-tailed it out of school before any rumbling had even started.

I was sitting at my desk when I saw a reflection of a flash of light on my laptop. *That's not what I think it is, is it?* I pretended that my eyelids had twitched or something. I kept typing, trying valiantly to focus on mapping out how I would teach the blues scale to my eighth graders.

Another short, quick flash against the computer screen. This time, it was followed a few seconds later by an insistent, low rumble. I froze, unable to move. *One one thousand, two one thousand, three one thousand . . .* My heart rate began to climb. My plan had been to work, then walk down the hill to catch the last bus to Riverdale. I couldn't do that now. I couldn't fathom walking through the dark campus, and then down an even darker, steep hill lined with massive, shadowy trees during this storm.

I stared at the computer screen, seeing nothing but the half-open window blinds and the dark outside beyond them. I focused intently on the alternating white-and-black stripes. My fingers stopped moving and the only sound in the room, in the entire building, was Miles Davis's "Freddie Freeloader" playing from the tiny speakers of the laptop. I waited, immobile, for the next bright flash, heart pumping in my throat and ears.

I missed the bus. I had been so focused on the potential horrors of walking to the bus stop that I lost track of time. Now I was screwed. How would I get home? *Fuck!* Although Masters was a boarding school and there would certainly be colleagues at home on campus, I was too embarrassed to call any of them. What would I say? "I'm scared of thunder, so can you drive me home?" or "Can I crash on your floor tonight because I'm a big baby?" My only option was to take the Metro-North to the Marble Hill station, and that walk would be even more terrifying. That train would leave in thirty minutes. *Mirna, think! Stop being such a fucking baby. It's just thunder. Just air expanding. It's only the angels bowling . . . You can do this.* While I was trembling, my eyes still glued to the screen, Bill the overnight security guard came by to lock up. Thank God. *Thank God.* I stood up and rushed toward him.

"Bill! Oh my God!" I began to sob and shake.

"Hey, hey, hey . . ." He came closer. "What's . . . what's the matter?"

"This is gonna sound really stupid, but I'm really afraid of thunder," I blurted.

"What . . . do you need me to sit here with you?" he asked sweetly.

Lightning exploded in the sky, this time with bolts that were discernible through the blinds. It looked like throbbing varicose veins.

"Will you drive me to the train station? Please? I just missed the last bus and I'm terrified of thunderstorms and I need to get home and I can't walk down there all alone. Please?" I asked, entire body trembling.

"Whoa. I mean, I don't know if I can leave campus."

"Bill, please? Please do me this favor." I closed my eyes and breathed in deeply. "Like, I'm really scared."

I think he realized that my fear was real. It was urgent and unreasonable.

"Um, okay, I guess I can do it." He was fairly new at the school and was probably worried he'd get in trouble. I didn't have the capacity to care about his job at this moment. I could only process my own fear, my own need to feel protected and safe.

He drove me to the station and, on the ride there, cracked jokes and reassured me that he would deliver me safely to the station. During the ride, the thunder subsided and the lightning flashes became fainter and more faded. I had only a few minutes until the train would come, and there were other folks waiting on the platform, so the shaking of my hands subsided a bit.

———

When I'm out running on the trail and there's a threat of a thunderstorm, my heart rate spikes, I start sweating profusely, my breathing becomes shallow, and I panic. My mind races: *Where should I go? Should I continue? Should I stop and hide under this tree?* Even on trail runs with no chance of a storm, I'm always on the hunt for hiding spots near rock outcroppings that could serve as potential thunder shelters.

Yeah, that one looks good, except for if there's a landslide, then that would suck. Ooh, look at that one. But it also looks like a den. A bear's den. And that one looks perfect, except for the fact that the lightning will probably strike this one because it's looking for me.

But I just keep going. Because *where else am I going to go?*

I've come to the realization that if I get electrocuted, then it was meant to happen.

If the loud thunder booms ruin my eardrums, then I'll just make like Beethoven and keep on living. If the tentacles of lightning decide to transport me into a *Close Encounters of the Third Kind* type of existence, well, so be it.

I take a deep breath to try to slow my breathing and heart rate and keep running or hiking. I continue to watch the sky darken and glance down every now and then so I don't fall flat on my face.

I can only keep going, knowing the storm will end at some point. It's up to me to carry on living and embodying and embracing the fear.

And then, magically, the storm will stop, and I will keep running.

13

The Agony and the Injury

Up until I started training for my first marathon, after I did a race, including the short ones (5Ks and 10Ks), I'd be sore for days. Sometimes my feet wouldn't stop hurting until the following 5K, and I just had to deal with the pain. Other times my legs barely functioned, but somehow, right before the next race, they magically unlocked so that I could finish the event. I usually came home with some kind of soreness or pain that would cause me to shuffle carefully, walk down the stairs backward, or limp imperceptibly. I didn't normally need to walk around in a clunky orthopedic boot, or on crutches, mind clouded by some heavy painkiller. Nope, not usually. But different circumstances call for different measures.

The summer of 2011 I was looking forward to running several races to prepare for what would be the big race of that season, the Marine Corps Marathon—my first attempt at running a marathon. One race was the North Face Endurance Challenge in Sterling, Virginia, which was set to happen two days after the Purnell School's graduation, allowing my friend Katie and me to hop in a car with our children; drive to Washington, DC; do the race; and hurry back to New Jersey so that we would be ready for our week of prettying up the campus for the alumnae reunion.

Early Saturday afternoon we were off, enjoying a longish ride to Alexandria, Virginia, where we would stay in her childhood home, listen to jazz, eat an excellent meal polished off with homemade rhubarb compote and ice cream, sleep deeply, and then nervously head over to what would be Katie's first half-marathon trail run. We were guaranteed excellent TNF swag, a beautiful course, and a race that had sufficient challenges to make it worth traveling a few hours in each direction.

I felt pretty good about my prospects of finishing within the cutoff, since I had completed the brutal (I thought) NJ Trail Series half marathon at Lewis Morris Park in Morristown a few weeks earlier in May, with a time of roughly 3:45:00. I was ready and excited to have traveled so far to run with a good friend (the one who would become responsible for introducing me to the ultramarathon gateway drug, the full marathon) on a new-to-me trail.

My only goal that day was to finish before the cutoff, which was a generous *four* hours, considering that most people are able to finish a half marathon in under three hours, many in under two. I had looked at the elevation profile beforehand, and surprisingly, it hadn't scared the shit out of me. There would be a couple of hills and valleys in the first few miles on this out-and-back course (it is a point-to-point course today, meaning it starts at one location and finishes in another), but it would flatten out and meander along the border between Virginia and Maryland along the Potomac River. The trail was primarily a single track with a short paved area in the beginning before it entered and quickly left a golf course to head into the lush forest lining the Potomac Heritage Trail.

Except for me, most of the runners were thin and competitive-looking, serious and focused, with furrowed brows and a slight air of je ne sais quoi. Most of the men wore running shorts with slits up the side, and many of the women had on short compression shorts or the kinds of shorts that I will never, ever be able to wear with my long, upside-down-trapezoid-shaped thighs. There was also a good share of nervous boasting à la I-did-such-and-such-marathon-at-such-and-such-altitude, blank stares, and a very long line for the Porta-Potties. I did a quick sweep of the runners lined up at the start, looking for the fat people. I scanned the crowd anxiously for any Clydesdale/Athena types who might also be taking the plunge with me.

I do this at every race: look for the fat people. I always wonder what their journey is and how it has been for them. I wonder what running means to them. Is it a means to lose weight? Are they intent on permanently changing or altering their physical and emotional lives? Did someone drag them here? And most importantly, will I be able to *pass* them and leave them in my own fat dust? I can be competitive too . . . though only at the end, when I know I won't have to exert any more energy, and if I need to collapse, at least it won't be in the middle of the race.

Well, there were no other curvies, Athenas, Clydesdales, or any other people who embodied a nontypical runner's body. Nope—just some taller, big-boned people who probably ran like gazelles and could consistently churn out eight-minute miles on a trail.

I lined up near the back of the pack, not kidding myself about my expected pace. I was hoping to maintain at least a fourteen-minute-per-mile pace, given that it was, you know, a *trail* race. The announcer counted down and we were off across the parking lot, down a hill, and onto the Potomac Heritage Trail. The first 1.5 miles were a breeze; at the beginning I run a little faster than normal because it's almost impossible not to, given the high adrenaline level of the entire crowd. It felt great! I was pretty far in the back, but not dead last and pretty confident that I would be able to pass some of the more smug runners. You know, the ones who go out entirely too fast and burn out by mile three. Still feeling pretty comfy, I ran through mildly technical sections on the trail, along with some absolutely gorgeous and peaceful single tracks.

I'm used to being in the back and running alone; this way, I don't have to pretend like I have enough breath control and cardio conditioning to hold a conversation with anyone. I run and enjoy being in nature while simultaneously listening to Ludacris, Nicki Minaj, Cat Stevens, and the Indigo Girls on my iPod. They help me pass a few struggling skinny runners. *A-ha!* I catch myself thinking mean thoughts—which I won't share.

Anyway, at around mile 3.5 a steep incline *came out of nowhere*, complete with annoying switchbacks. *Ugh. Okay, I still got this, right?* I had already passed about four people, so I was feeling a little smug. I had done a lot of hill work with my cross-country girls in the spring, so although the hills were still difficult, I didn't feel as though I was dying. I kept a steady power-hiking pace and got to the top. And then I started the series of steep descending switchbacks. It felt awesome to power-run down the descent, leaving yet another runner in my fat dust! I felt like a fat super.

And then, *without* falling, I rolled the outside of my left ankle a good ninety degrees.

Somehow I did not fall. Perhaps I owe it to all the core-strengthening exercises I had been doing during the spring to help me remain mostly upright. I hobbled a bit, in shock from the intense pain that followed the very loud popping sound.

"Wow, I *heard* that," said the man I had passed about two-tenths of a mile back. I slid down the nearest tree trunk and sat down on the rocky slope, wincing and cursing. *Fuuccckkk!* He looked at the ankle and said he didn't see anything sticking out, so I should be good. This is how we trail runners do. He then continued on. This too was my plan.

I got up, which was a long and laborious process. The throbbing from my ankle made my entire body pulsate sympathetically, painfully. *This is bad,* I thought. Other times, when I have slipped on wet leaves, or slammed my big toe against a plainly visible rock or branch, I have found it relatively easy to get back up and limp a little—eventually the pain would subside. But this time was strikingly different. I had to roll over onto my knees, grab the tree trunk, and then hop onto my right leg without putting any pressure on the left foot. The throbbing worsened. The first step was excruciatingly painful, the next a little less so, and the third was I-can-get-to-the-next-aid-station-if-I-limp-really-fast painful. I hobbled for a little over a mile, still mostly downhill, until I reached the aid station. The guy who had passed me had alerted them to my condition.

On my way to that aid station, I toyed with the idea of DNFing. *Should I stop at the aid station and wait for the medics to take me back to the start? Should I try to finish this even if it takes me four hours? Should I sit down and cry? Should I stand here and click my heels three times?* (Well, no, that would incur more pain, so that was out of the question!) *Should I try to finish? Should I try to finish? Should I try to finish?*

And then I imagined the scene back at the finish area: me being helped out of the medic's ATV. Fat girl limping.

No thanks.

I had to do this for fat people. I had to do this for me. And I had to finish because I didn't want *anybody* thinking that the fat girl couldn't do it.

I arrived at the aid station. The volunteers were ready for me.

"Do you want us to get the medics out here?"

Hell no! "I'd love some Advil if you have any." I took three pills, retied my shoelaces, and went about my way. A few minutes later, I was able to limp-run-walk-hop, wincing less and less as the miles went by slowly. I tried not to think of the beating pain from the ankle and tried to focus instead on staying ahead of a woman I had passed a long time ago who was now gaining on me.

At a crucial juncture on the course, she passed me as I was taking a break. Later I passed her again at a wide spot on the trail. Then she passed me and blocked my way on the single track back to the finish for about two miles. She wouldn't budge. I was right on her tail, but didn't have it in me to say "To your left" or "To your right." *Okay, missy. I got this.* I stayed right on her heels until we reached a wider part of the trail. She stopped to take a break. I took the opportunity to pass her without ever looking back. You can only imagine the string of expletives that oozed out of my mouth.

Mile ten came and went, and the pain in my ankle began to ramp up, but the only thought I had was *This woman isn't that far behind me, so I can't get off pace too much even if I'm in pain.* (I know, I can be stupid and vain. I'm well aware.) I slowed down just a bit to guzzle tepid Gatorade. There were still about 1.7 miles to go, so I walked until I heard the people at the last aid station start to cheer. I looked back, only to see that woman gaining on me.

And then, like something out of a made-for-TV drama, I screamed *"Nooooooooooooooo!"* as if the film was suddenly blurry and in slow motion. I hobbled-ran-walked-hopped-skipped-limped as fast as I could to the end, this time because I was *mad*, and I certainly wasn't going to let this woman get ahead of me and gloat that she wasn't last. *She* was going to be last—the fat girl wouldn't be.

I gathered enough energy—*adrenaline is crack*—to run through the finishing chute, raising the roof.

Now I could visit the medics on my own terms.

———

The following week back at work, the faculty had been charged with organizing and staffing the alumnae reunion, which always fell the week after graduation. Each person had different tasks: some of us moved furniture, some prepared linens for the dorm rooms, and others set up twinkling lights in the trees surrounding the main quad where most of the former students, faculty, and their families would be congregating. I was on the twinkling-lights team.

I was wearing a pair of flip-flops because my left ankle had been so swollen that I couldn't fit into any other shoe. I shuffled, hobbled, and limped about to the sympathetic and concerned looks of my colleagues—all except for my good friend Robin, who was also tasked with hanging lights. She sneered at me.

"What the hell are you doing?" she asked me.

"I'm fucking hanging lights like I'm supposed to," I said, annoyed. I knew what she was getting at.

"You can barely walk. And you're wearing flip-flops. What the *hell* is wrong with you?"

"I'm fine."

"You *clearly* are not."

"I sprained my ankle. Like, seriously it's not a big deal," I said.

"You 'sprained' your ankle *four* days ago. If it was a sprain, it wouldn't be so swollen. I mean, that thing is so swollen. Goddammit, I'm calling my orthopedist."

"Robin! I'm fine. You don't have to . . ." But before I could stop her, she was on her cell phone, making an appointment. For me.

"Eleven thirty tomorrow. Now, let's get you wrapped up. I can't believe you're walking around like this."

———

After surviving a series of cringe- and yelp-inducing movements for which I was told to bend my foot this way and that, the doctor smiled a tight smile that portended bad news.

"Well, the good news is that it's not *completely* broken," she said cheerfully. "It's called an avulsion fracture. When you twisted your ankle, your tendon ripped off a piece of bone."

"So what's the, um, *bad* news?" I asked, my shoulders deflating in anticipation for the moment when she told me I wouldn't be able to run the Marine Corps Marathon in the fall and that I probably wouldn't be able to ever run again.

"You'll be able to do your marathon," she said. I breathed a sigh of relief.

"But you won't be able to run for another eight weeks," she added. "You can pick up training then. You have a lot of miles on your legs already, so as long as you keep up your fitness regimen, you'll be able to do it. In about six weeks you'll be able to get on the elliptical and maybe a bike. And then we'll see. Until then, it's swimming, swimming, and more swimming, but only after the swelling has gone down and you're in almost no pain."

Ugh! What was I going to do? I trusted the doctor because she was also a runner and she understood how important finishing a marathon was for me. I had told her my whole story, about how I had thought I was having a heart attack years before and how running helped me achieve a whole new level of fitness that I hadn't had since high school. I cried a bit in the office, worried that I wouldn't really be able to do the full marathon.

June, July, and most of August that summer, I was most unpleasant to be around. In fact, I was so grumpy that my personal trainer, Mary, told me so.

"You're *miserable*," she said, grimacing and wrinkling her brow. I was on the elliptical machine doing nonimpact exercise, frowning, and complaining. It was the only machine I could be on, since my left ankle had *just* returned to its normal size after having been swollen, discolored, and tender for the preceding four weeks. My orthopedist had allowed me to start doing non-weight-bearing exercise, and I could do one elliptical session a week, as long as I didn't have any pain.

"Okay, off," Mary said. She was younger than I and had a baby face that belied her physical strength and confidence. She knew what she was doing.

"Thank God," I said, sighing. Nikki, who was on the machine next to me, snickered and then full-out laughed.

Mary took me through a series of gentle ankle-flexibility exercises. They were painful, but I trusted in her knowledge and wisdom. She was also a physical therapist.

Even though I was back at it, I wasn't *running*. In fact, I couldn't run because if I did, I'd probably be prolonging the injury that *some people* thought I had brought on myself, simply by choosing to continue running on that trail. Nikki was on the elliptical next to me, barely able to hide her laughing, rolling her eyes in an I-told-you-so kind of way. This had *obviously* been my fault.

The eight weeks of recovery and slow reentry into running were agonizing. I could handle the pain of the fractured ankle, and even the inability to rotate and bend it for weeks. Hell, I had run and walked the remaining nine miles of the TNF Endurance Challenge half marathon on it, right? That was the easy part. The hardest part was the inability to run. That movement had helped me change the direction of my life; it was the activity that jump-started my mornings and afternoons, that introduced me to a whole new community of friends, the reason I was able to physically withstand punishingly long days at work. Running allowed me to become a better person in general. And now I couldn't do it.

Seeing people out running on the hilly roads by school made me nostalgic and angry. After I could move about without the ugly boot, I slowly returned to my gym routine. I frequented yoga classes, and the pool became my best friend. I spent the bulk of my time running back and forth in the pool lanes after I had swum the requisite thirty minutes. Sometimes, the pain would come back, fierce and insistent, and I would have to sit or lie down with my foot elevated. Other times, I felt completely normal and pain-free. Seven weeks after the initial doctor's visit, I was able to lightly run (hidden of course, and without my doctor's release . . . but

I was so close!) on the soft trail of our cross-country course. My mojo was returning, and my bitterness toward the world began to subside. I stopped throwing angry eye-darts at other runners and obsessing over how many weeks of training I had lost.

In reality, I had actually become stronger. Cross-training became a necessity, and so I focused on strength and endurance in other areas. I could swim for more than an hour and ride the elliptical for an equal amount of time. I lifted weights, worked on flexibility with Mary, and learned how to modify exercises so that I wouldn't further damage my foot. So when my orthopedist finally released me, I went straight into training on an abbreviated schedule with only a few weeks of long runs before embarking on my first marathon, jumping right into thirteen miles that weekend. I knew immediately that I would make it to Marine Corps.

14

Do the Work

People always ask me how I get through those long, interminable miles during a race and how the hell I survive weekend after weekend of putting training miles in on road and trail. I don't have a magic pill or a quick fix. It's as simple as putting the work in, day in and day out.

In fact, nature has such a profound effect on me that I could keep moving my body through it for an eternity (unless it's one of those times when I get spooked for some reason). On those days when I'm in nature, I feel the most invigorated and alive. My step is light, my mind is calm, and I'm in a zone filled with calm, limitless energy brimming right under my skin. My big feet fit effortlessly in the grooves of a technical trail. The pebbles and larger rocks that play Hide-and-Seek with me under soft and crunchy leaves in autumn hues do so whimsically. I begin to feel like a parkour expert stepping easily from some deep grove to the top of a boulder in a rock garden, and then gracefully hopping off, landing soundlessly on the giving ground. I become the trail and the trail becomes me. I see the moon . . .

I have experienced deep, sublime moments while out on both trail and road. Once, my friend Rebecca and I ran nine miles in the hot northern Georgia sun the day after the Charleston shooting of nine people. We felt no pain and no hardship as our bodies and minds quietly honored those who had succumbed to the shooter's evil intentions.

Once, I found myself running alone on the deserted snow-covered trails of my school's cross-country course on a snow day, flakes landing softly on my nose.

Another time I ran in the cool, crisp Tongass National Forest in Alaska on trails framed by jagged snow-covered mountains in the distance. Time was of no concern. I had nary a worry, and my brow was furrowed only by the intensity of the sun's rays in my face.

And then there was the time when I finished my first marathon, with pain rolling in waves all over my body. The elation I felt as I crossed the finish line of the Marine Corps Marathon, high-fiving two marines. *Oorah!*

All these moments are, of course, tempered by the times I spend wondering why the hell I'm doing this because it's so damn hard, or because it hurts, or because I could be recovering from a tough week at work on the couch. In the middle of a hot and hilly 20-miler on a technical trail, sometimes I have to remind myself that I *chose* to do this, and I *chose* to surrender myself to the ever-changing topography and whims of nature. I *chose* to put on those clothes that rubbed a hole in my thigh. I *chose* to wear shoes that wouldn't protect my big toes those times I stubbed them against those same rocks and boulders that were playing Hide-and-Seek earlier. I *chose* a 50K over thirteen miles. I made all those choices.

Nobody ever achieved anything epic without doing the requisite work, even if the work itself is humdrum, boring, run-of-the-mill kind of work. Getting your weekly miles in, doing cross-training to strengthen your muscles and lessen the likelihood of overuse injuries, (for some) having a stretching/yoga regimen, eating to fuel (and enjoy life), and taking rest and recovery seriously (I admit that I haven't always done this) are all part of getting the work done.

I once wrote on Facebook, "Boy does marathon training take over your life." And this post was true. I traded in—well, I don't really know what I traded in because I can't for the life of me remember what I did before I started all this long-distance stuff. I guess I traded in early mornings for extremely early mornings. I normally woke up at five anyway to get in a couple of miles while I binge-watched every season of *Drop Dead Diva*, a show that strived to be different from other shows by featuring a smart, successful, larger-bodied person in a positive, non-matronly, and attractive role. Unfortunately, the show still employed the tired trope of the pretty, dumb blonde and her various male-finding exploits. I watched it anyway because, when I needed it to, it took my mind away from the hour or so that I would be spending on the tread-mill or the Spin bike. It also boosted my confidence as I slaved away on the hamster wheel.

———

When I started marathon training, three times a week my day would begin at four so I could inhale some joe, chew on a piece of dry toast with peanut butter, and rush out of the house to drive the twenty or so dark miles to Berkeley Heights, New Jersey, that housed what was quickly becoming my second home, Life Time Athletic club.

That gym was unlike any other gym in which I had ever been a member. It was open twenty hours a day with a variety of classes that I enjoyed immensely and that started before six in the morning. I loved the instructors and their commitment to holistic health. I loved the fact that I felt like people were watching and lauding my progress, not just in weight loss but also in endurance and strength. This gym also had phenomenal coffee. I was sold!

My workouts usually followed a similar routine: I ran a few miles to warm up and worked to fulfill the weekly mileage or time on my feet that was required by Jenny Hadfield and John Bingham's *Marathoning for Mortals* training plan. I then did a boot-camp or interval class for an hour, an hour in which I would simultaneously berate myself for not being able to do a million-plus-one burpees and thoroughly enjoy myself being a part of the living-and-breathing organism of that class. The instructor walked around and cracked jokes about everyone, liberally, without missing a count. He knew all the regulars and what they were doing with their training. The same three women arrived fifteen minutes early and laid down their mats, weights, resistance bands (always the red ones!), and step platforms (they used *three*, dammit!) right in the front. They also complained loudly if the class started thirty seconds late or if the pace of the music wasn't fast enough for them. They never, ever missed a class unless our instructor, DeWayne, had called out sick and some other instructor, who was *clearly* incompetent according to their disgusted and dissatisfied body language and tongue clicking, was leading. One of them had a perm and looked like she was straight out of the '80s with her stacked socks or leggings. She was also extremely thin, and I caught myself wondering from time to time why in the hell she would need to take this class. (I know, unfair, but she was especially cranky and impatient, so I'm allowing myself this bit of disdain.) She was the most annoying of the trio, sneering and looking askance at people she perceived as slowing down the class. *Pipe down, bitch!* was a frequently occurring thought.

After this class, I headed down to the heated pool and swam laps for half an hour. I emerged from the pool drenched, feeling heavy and satisfied, only to submerge myself immediately in the cascading waterfall of the hot whirlpool, willing the soreness in my muscles to both stay and go away.

I showered each morning in the luxuriously appointed locker room, lathering myself generously in the fancy mint-smelling bodywash and lotion, taking my time to dress for work. I then bought the largest coffee available and headed back home to get Rashid ready for school if

Cito hadn't already and then headed to work, ready and energized . . . and smelling minty.

School began at eight o'clock in the morning and ended at 3:30 p.m. Because I lived on campus, I sometimes snuck home to get in a second workout on the treadmill or bike when I had a planning period. When I say I went all in, I mean it: *I. Went. All. In.* Few things were more important than making sure that I had done all the work I needed to do to continue on my clearly successful path to vastly improved health and wellness.

In the evenings after school, I did exercise videos. My favorites were any of the *Biggest Loser* videos because they were challenging workouts with people, some of whom resembled me, of different shapes and sizes. They didn't idealize thin people nor were they condescending to fat people in an obvious way, unless you count the time when Jillian Michaels kept mentioning one of the contestants' big JLo booty. *Come on, really?* Other than that, I learned new exercises to incorporate into my routine, and I became stronger and even more motivated to attain another level of fitness.

The big change in lifestyle occurred on the weekends. Generally, on Saturdays I allowed myself to sleep in until five. After waking up, I consumed enough calories to sustain me through the first five or so miles of my long run, and then I headed out to a local trail or dirt road to put in the work.

The issue wasn't the long mileage. The issue was what happened afterward. I often felt okay for the first few minutes after finishing a long run (I quickly learned that I needed to eat, drink, and keep moving) until my heart rate returned to normal, but then fierce leg cramps would start, along with a new level of fatigue I had never encountered. My big flat feet hurt, and that pain would take days to lessen. My back and shoulders became sore, as would my core, and other muscles in my body that I had no idea existed for the purpose of running. For some relief, I lay down on the couch, immobile for hours afterward. I was useless.

———

One of my favorite events is the Catamount Ultra in Stowe, Vermont, with its two options: the 25K or the 50K. I like to do the 25K because the following week is another of my favorite races, the Finger Lakes 50s 50K. Even though I know that I'm in for some difficult running and lots of power-hiking up steep hills in the Green Mountains, I've put in the requisite work to at least finish the mileage, alive, standing (barely), and renewed mentally, even if finishing means I must suffer through fatigue and temporary pain to keep finding ways to move my body through nature.

I did this race for the first time in June of 2015 after having stalked the website for more than a year. *Would I be able to do it? What was the cutoff, and would I make it?* Probably too short and probably no. *Would I be the only black person there?* Likely. *Would I be the only fat person there?* Most likely.

Despite all my questions, the answers were an invitation for me to get my ass up there and continue showing the world that people who aren't white/male/skinny/athletic-looking, et cetera can participate in these types of events and even be successful, provided that they're dedicated to the months of preparation needed to at least get to the start line.

This particular course is a fairly difficult one, with a climb totaling 2,500 feet per loop of 15.5 miles. To a mountain climber that elevation might sound, say, easy. I'm not a mountain climber. However, I do love my trails to be interesting and rolling. The first six miles of the Catamount is a net uphill.

I knew going into it that it would be a slog, pretty much from the first mile in with a couple (read: *a few*) coastable downhills, "flat" sections, and tolerable rolling hills that you can't get yourself through using momentum built up from short downhills. I knew that the first 10K would be really tough and that it would probably not be enjoyable. I knew that my legs would hurt and that at times I would feel as if I were only utilizing half a lung, if that.

I also knew that there would be sweeping views of the gently sloping Green Mountains, encounters with *Is-that-a-moose-or-a-bear-or-a-tree?* There would be the downhills that would instantly throw me into the flow zone, allowing me to forget the vert that just happened. Some say childbirth is extremely painful but that you forget the pain as soon as you're healed. That wasn't my experience during labor and the birth of my son, and yet I never, ever wanted to experience that shit again. But long-distance trail running must be the runner-up to the whole childbirth experience—many times it's painful and extremely exhausting, and sometimes you do actually think *I am never doing this fucking shit again. Why the fuck did I sign up for this shit? I'm dying. No, for real. I'm dying. Why do I keep doing this to myself?* But after it's over, I want to do it again. And again. As soon as you hit those flats, or the non-quad-crushing gently sloping downhills, you forget that you left your lung up at the top of that hill. You forget that you also left your knees and ankles there too. You forget that you were ever contemplating throwing yourself into the ravine, because that's a way-easier route—maybe more painful in the end, but easier *right now.*

When I run ultramarathon courses like the Catamount Ultra, I have my strategies to deal with the hills. Sometimes you just look at a hill and say, "Okay, let's be friends. Let's do this, dammit!" And then you do it. Quickly power-hiking or prancing up it like those crazy-fast folks who never seem to tire while working themselves up hill after hill, their dusty and muddy calf muscles streaked with sweat, the only sign of exertion. Their faces, locked in a neutral but determined expression, belie the actual heart-pounding effort required to skip lightly and unobtrusively over rocks, small boulders, ditches, and grooves. These people make no sound, like special agents in the military. They sneak up on you, light of foot, easily whizzing by your lumbering, heavy body that is gasping for air on every lead-footed step, the sweat running liberally down your face, stinging your eyes and dampening your already malodorous technical apparel that will dry in the sun and then smell some more.

Sometimes you look at a hill, feeling fatigued and resenting that you have placed yourself at the mercy of the natural contour of the earth yet again. Some force other than your intellectual self signed you up for this. Some fleeting whimsy held you and your credit card hostage while it quickly filled in a mostly prepopulated form that already knew your T-shirt size. And now here you are, standing at the foot of an enormous, rocky hill—maybe at the foot of Mount Mansfield in Vermont, maybe near the end of an already hilly half-marathon trail in the southern Appalachians, or maybe at the foot of the Brooklyn Bridge.

You might ask: *Why do this? What is the reward?*

For each hill you conquer—rather, *take* (because no one can conquer nature)—you receive a reward of momentary relief, which can fuel another few miles. Maybe you get a brief respite before the next hill or switchback. Perhaps you're blessed with a view of a far-off mountain range with rock faces jutting out perfectly against a cloudless sky like your own private Everest. Maybe you come upon a partially obstructed view of a sparkling mountain lake or river. Maybe the rustle of trees in the too-warm, too-humid but suddenly breezy air cools you for a bit. Perhaps . . .

Sometimes, you receive no reward, no prize for your efforts, except for the fact that you're able and willing to put forth the effort and do the work to slog up this hill and others that will certainly come after.

Like many runners, I do the work because I can, and there is honor in that. Honoring my body, honoring the sport. Honoring my family that allows me to train endlessly on weekends when I could/should be attending basketball games, socializing with my book group, planning and making elaborate "clean" meals, sleeping in with my spouse, running errands . . . Honoring the human body by moving through nature as it is meant to do.

Sometimes, though, getting out the door takes an eternity for what I'm supposed to be doing. I hit "Snooze" on all three of my alarms and grab an extra minute or two between buzzes and beeps. I roll over and complain silently about how sore my legs are or how I need coffee to even get out of bed.

Interestingly enough, as soon as I make the decision to get out of bed, which I typically need to do on a daily basis anyway (you know, child, work, self-care, that sort of thing), tasks become much easier. The less I think about what I have to do—two miles on the track, a frigid three miles at thirteen degrees, some "speed" work on my creaky and loud treadmill, a cross-training workout, yoga session, or whatever I have planned for the day—the more doable and enjoyable it is after I get over myself. I have only to get dressed and go.

But then I encounter the counter with all its mail to organize, lesson plans to rework, books to read, blog-post ideas to outline from brainstorms scribbled on random scraps of paper and sticky notes. I have to brew my strong black coffee and make several bathroom trips. Oh, and the weekly post for *Women's Running Magazine* to write, and that mountain of bills to pay, that form to sign for Rashid's something or other, the long list of college recommendations to write, the school books to order, the millions of undone, unchecked-off items on my imaginary to-do list to accomplish.

But I have to run. I know that if I don't run in the morning, I'll have only limited opportunity in the afternoon or evening. If I don't run, I will perseverate about it all day, thinking and talking about it constantly. My son will notice a change in my demeanor: "Mom, did you run (or work out) this morning? Because you're, like, really cranky."

So I drink the coffee, scalding my tongue every morning. I put on my snazzy running clothes (the only articles of clothing in my closet that live up to that adjective), including my fancy compression socks, my shoes (different according to how long I'll be running, and whether on track, trail, road, or treadmill), and a bra that will hold the ladies in place long enough so I don't get a bruised chin or chest. I then step out onto the lawn/drive to the gym/head to my guest room/turn on an exercise video/put on my Pitbull, Indigo Girls, Stevie Wonder, Puccini, Daddy Yankee, Drake, Cranberries, Ani DiFranco, Brahms playlists, and then I start.

My heart rate rises and settles after a few minutes at a higher comfortable-but-not-doable-forever rate, my feet find their footing easily, my arms swing too high, my heavy head hangs too low, my headlamp offers a distorted view of a few feet ahead on the track, spotted with goose poop. I listen for the birds that sound like baby horses in the dark. I hear coyotes in the distance on cold winter mornings. I watch my breath; I notice the particles in the air through the dense fog, the humidity rising from the wet or frozen grass of the soccer field.

Nothing is more pleasurable than this work, this run.

15

THEY CALLED ME COACH

"Way to go, coach! Nice job!" said Dan, the athletic director at the Purnell School.

Did he just call me coach? I thought. *Wait, did he really? No one's ever called me that before. I mean, I know I'm a coach, but . . . Wow, I'm a* coach*!*

That late October afternoon in 2010 had turned bitterly cold and dark. Three girls who needed to be picked up were still out on the gravel of McCann Mill Road near Pottersville, New Jersey. Luckily, they were only about a half mile away from school, so they still earned the right to say they had finished the longest run of their short lives thus far.

I had already finished with a few girls who had initially doubted they could even do *half* the distance I asked them to do for our last cross-country practice. It was our capstone run, so to speak. Most of them finished with a solid nine miles under their belts, and for those who had to be picked up, their mileage still surpassed anything they had ever done. There were Morgan, Maddy, Hannah, Anna, Cathy, and Jiaming—a veritable mix of cultures, abilities, and experience with athleticism. Many of them had never run or participated in any other sport before.

They were all students at the Purnell School, a small all-girls boarding school located in the part of Jersey that most New Yorkers (like myself, I must admit) didn't even know existed. Trees and shit, cow farms, and silos. It was my third year at the school, and my life had already started to change in significant ways. Running and other fitness-related activities had taken over most every aspect of my nonteaching and nonfamily life. I would leave school during a break and run on the local paved bike trail just south in Bedminster. I would schedule my entire weekend around long runs, classes at the gym, and local races. I even once told a half-truth to one of my colleagues. I needed to run an errand—an errand that happened to be at the gym a half an hour away. (Well, I was technically *running*, just on a treadmill . . .) People began to take notice of my running habit. I was slowly losing some of the protracted adiposity around my midsection, and I looked and felt more radiant and healthy than I had since my son was born. Dan, also a brilliantly funny history teacher, caught me at a moment when I couldn't contain my enthusiasm and good karma from running. I had to share it.

"So, um, wanna go for a run tomorrow with me and the girls?" I asked Nikki, the day before our epic last run.

"How long? I don't trust you. You'll say five and then we'll end up doing ten. How long?" She exaggerated her words. "So I can mentally prepare to die."

"Just nine—"

"Nine?" she repeated, loudly and in her raspy, high voice. "You're trying to kill me, right?" She shook her head.

"Precisely. We meet at three thirty in front of the—"

"I know, I know." She walked away shaking her head and mumbling, "I don't know how I let you talk me into this. Incredible."

Nikki would be out in the front with the faster girls, and another colleague I recruited, Sandy, would be midpack. I would be in the back, bringing up the rear. We set off from the school gym at around four, when the temperature had dipped to just below mild and the sun had started its slow fade in Central Jersey, behind the rolling hills of cow and horse pastures, expansive estates, and requisite country clubs.

I had run this course countless times in my own training. In fact, it was my favorite. I knew every dip in the road, where there might be a deer crossing, where the elderly man might be on his daily walk with his infirm canine companion. The run started at our school campus and went across a bridge over the beautiful and clear, smooth-rock-bottomed Black River, down an almost two-mile stretch of dirt-and-gravel road with an occasional house on either side, across the Lamington River, down a windy stretch of exposed road until it hit a section of road to Oldwick that was composed primarily of hills. Both sides of the road were framed with picturesque horse farms, stately homes that weren't quite mansions (but longed to be), and Holstein cow pastures. The turnaround point was at the Oldwick General Store that served what were likely the best deli sandwiches (salami and provolone on a roll, with mayo, oil and vinegar, and "seasoning") and lemonade in Central Jersey. On my own long runs, I often stopped there to use the bathroom, grab a steamy black coffee, and chew on some Tootsie Rolls prior to heading back home or adding a few more hilly miles before returning.

This day was special. I was preceded and trailed by a total of about fifteen girls, who would embark on their first-ever run above six miles. It wasn't a competitive team (we didn't run meets), but we trained like one. We had put in the requisite work: short runs, medium-length runs, long runs, cross-training, optional boot camps, interval training, and local 5K races on the weekends. We ran in extreme heat, wind, and cold. I made them run in cold rain. Sometimes members of the team ran before dawn, joining me in my daily morning workouts around a mile-long, unlit loop of houses near school. They were ready, both physically and mentally, even if some of them doubted they'd be able to finish in the beginning.

I found myself saying things like "Trust your training," "It's just another mile," "Run until that car goes over the hill and then take a break," and "Do you wanna miss dinner?"

I had bought a bunch of energy gels and water bottles for the occasion and deposited them about 2.5 miles in so that the girls could carry them to the turnaround point and experience the miracle that is GU.

And like a drug dealer, I told them to "Just trust me; this stuff works. *Trust me.*"

"Ms. Valerio, it's like, it's . . . it's magic," said Morgan.

"I know. It's a little gross at first (and at last), but it gives you, like, new life, right? *I know.*"

Morgan proceeded to blast all of us out of the water, finishing her run in about an hour and a half (fast for our group)!

The rest of us slowpokes walked and ran, chatting and challenging each other to run up this hill, power-hike that one, run this flat until the pole, sprint until the herd of cows, run until the cars disappear so we don't look like we're being lazy, catch up to Ms. B (Nikki), or don't let so-and-so pass you, let's make it look like this is easy . . .

When we got to the turnaround point, we watered ourselves, boosted our energy stores with GU, Clif Bloks, and Tootsie Rolls, then reconfigured and set out to complete the second half of our expedition.

Two miles away from the finish, some of the girls became fatigued, doubtful that they would be able to finish.

"Hey, ladies, how's it going?"

"Ms. Valerio, I'm cold," said Maddy.

"And my legs hurt, like really bad," said Jiaming.

Both girls shuffled stiffly.

"Trust your training," I said. "You're tired? I am too. But we've got to get back, right? We can't stand here and be cold. Let's go and get this done. Forward!"

"Um, okay," Maddy said softly. Jiaming moved forward silently.

The slowdown was painful to watch. You could see the strain in their faces as they climbed up just one more hill and tried to will their legs where their minds and spirits were. They knew that just one or two more pushes would elicit success.

It was getting even darker and colder. Most of us hadn't prepared for that. I was in capris, a T-shirt, and a light running jacket, which would have been fine had I been running, um, faster.

"Ladies, you got this. If I can do this, then you can do it too. We've all trained for this moment. We've done the work, in the cold, in the heat, and in the rain. We can do this, okay? Are you listening?"

"Yes, Ms. Valerio . . . but it's so cold, and I can't feel my hands," Maddy said.

"Then keep moving." Tough sell, but they obliged.

The cold penetrated my bones so much that it was hard to move and believe in my own motivational words. But it was my job to inspire them to keep going, and the practice was good for me too. It got me out of my own head and taught me to place the needs of my team before my own. After that, it became almost easy. The energy I had spent worrying about whether my own fingers would fall off was replaced by this new kind of energy. I had done the run before many times, so I knew *I* could do it. Now there was this matter of whether I could motivate my girls to finish something we had all at one point thought was impossible.

I ran up and down the last stretch of dirt road that was becoming the spooky dark that is just south of the last light but not completely dark . . . you know, the creepy crepuscular light that makes it difficult to see everything because your eyes don't know whether to adjust to darkness or hope for light. I had to make sure the last girls were still moving. I couldn't leave them out there, so I kept myself warm by running to and from them.

Finally, it became almost too dark to see—there were no street lamps or anything to speak of (we *were* in horse country). Just when I had that thought, Marcia, who had already finished her portion of the run, drove by. She rolled down her window and the warm air from her silver Volkswagen Passat hit my face, inviting me to shorten my run.

"You guys okay? I just wanted to check up on the girls."

"I'm okay, but I think Maddy and Jiaming are done. They will still have eight and a half miles under their belts, which is the longest either of them has ever run. I call it a win. So yeah, um, can you take them back?" Puffs of steam came out of my mouth whenever I talked.

I felt bad for them. Both girls had been excited and nervous about this day, and true to both of their work ethics, they had done everything I had asked of them to prepare.

I finished the run to the school and headed immediately to the dining hall. Faculty members who lived on campus were required to eat at assigned tables with the students, so I went straight to mine, not noticing the applause that had erupted when I entered. I was the last person to finish.

They were applauding for our cross-country girls and their accomplishment. They were also recognizing me, their coach.

As we stood in preparation for grace, Dan came by, patted me on the back, and said "Way to go, coach. Nice job!" The soccer coach, William (whose wife, Kathy, had driven me to the ER two years prior), also chimed in, "Nice job, coach!"

I'll always connect the meal that evening to that moment in the dining hall. The German-themed dinner included cabbage and apples, spicy pork chops braised in sauerkraut, colorful roasted root vegetables, and potato pancakes served with applesauce and sour cream.

We were congratulated during announcements at dinner, and the community clapped and wooted for us again. They were likely tired of my daily reminders during lunch that *yes, we will be running today, in the rain—unless there is a tornado or hurricane. We will be on the road. Running. And please don't ask me what we're doing today, because the answer is going to be the same thing every day. Every. Day. Running.*

They called me *coach*.

This is one of the highest honors that, as an educator, has been bestowed upon me. I hadn't really considered myself a coach yet, because when I started with the girls, I was still learning how to train and coach *myself* into shape for my own upcoming marathon. I had to educate myself about periodization—structuring training in a series of micro- and macrocycles, the purpose and benefits of long runs, speed work, cross-training, and endurance-sports nutrition.

I was also still working furiously on losing weight (which I continue to do) and trying desperately to maintain energy stores while becoming a marathoner. I had to adhere to my own training and complement it with or incorporate it into the training plan I had for my girls.

However, sometimes I had to put my own training needs aside. When my own plan called for four miles and the girls were suffering from heat fatigue or dehydration, I didn't always get what I needed done. I had to make amends, be flexible, and run on the treadmill in my apartment between classes, and compromise by adding mileage to my next run or skipping a run entirely. I eventually learned how to balance my runs and theirs, and as I coached more, I was able to anticipate when I would need to move things around in my own schedule.

During the late summer of 2010, as I stood in line to pay for my organic maple-walnut bread at the local farmers' market one Saturday morning, Dan approached me and asked if I wanted to make a couple hundred dollars extra by taking some girls on my runs after school.

I was sold. I was going to run most days anyway, so why not take some girls along with me? Yes. That was an easy answer.

And that's how my coaching started. It would be a natural extension of my somewhat unorthodox teaching methods and yet another valuable way in which to get to know my students more deeply outside of the Spanish classes and diversity seminar that Nikki and I had developed.

I was full of nerves the first day of practice. Would the girls take me seriously? I mean, I didn't *look* the part of a running coach. Would *I* be able to keep up with *them*? Would I embarrass myself? Would they make fun of my weird gait and my jiggling fat? Mind you, I have no problem making a complete fool of myself—it's par for the course as a teacher—but I still had a niggling concern that this whole coaching thing would be a bust.

None of that happened. Most of the students were happy to be able to try the sport without judgment and without fear of being cut or counseled out and encouraged to do something that required less coordination. They were girls who had decided to attend the school for these precise reasons. The classes were small and intimate, and we teachers lived in the dorms with them, coached them, and chaperoned trips with them on the weekends. It was an intense but loving environment. Those girls were our family, and we were theirs. They trusted us with their anxieties and insecurities, and we learned much about them and ourselves in turn. It's likely the unique environment at Purnell allowed me to be creative in coaching so that I frequently receive Facebook messages and e-mails like this:

> I honestly couldn't have asked for a better coach. Your honesty was so relaxing to be around. While any other time I was coached in XC it was very much competition oriented, I learned a whole new point of view of xc with you. I feel like running with you was so much more about doing something that made you feel good and have fun, and bond with the people you were with. No one felt embarrassed to have to take a break or walk. It was an absolutely judgment-free zone and I loved that! And we were

always laughing and having fun! It was very thera-
peutic and a perfect way to end the day. While we
were having fun you also were very inspiring the
way you would push yourself. You were the first to
want to go up that steep hill! And we would all join
in. Being coached by someone that you can tell
genuinely enjoys the run and is pushing themselves
right beside you was so amazingly unique, and created such a positive and open environment.

Another student who recently graduated from college wrote:

As a senior in high school the last thing on my
mind was an hour of sport requirements I had to
fill. I had joined cross-country on a whim. I thought,
eh, running can't be that hard, and gave it a try.
Being heavier myself at the time I had no motivation to work out or change my lifestyle. I remember
the first day of the winter season we were told to
run up the sports fields, behind them, and finish
the loop around to the gym. I only got to the first
sports field when I realized this new hobby I took
up was going to kick my ass. Not only did it do that,
but it ultimately became an outlet.

Ms. Valerio changed my view on exercise completely. It was hard since it was cold, you could
feel it in your lungs, which even made it hard to
breathe. Every step of the way she was there to run
with us, encourage us and motivate us. By finding
new routes to run and activities she always made it
different. What felt like an impossible loop around

the campus soon became my favorite way to spend the days. It was hard and I would often run out of breath, but Ms. Valerio was there to tell me it wasn't going to be easy but just a little farther every day really does make the difference. She made a runner out of a big doubter. Even on days when it would rain and snow she set up indoor obstacles and exercises to keep us in the groove.

On weekends she even offered to take students on different 5Ks in the area. Finally when spring came around I felt as if I was ready, I had never done a race before but I was able to complete it without stopping. Ms. Valerio always had a passion for running and had a great way of passing that on to her students. For me, running started out as a way to fill my sports requirement but soon was an outlet. I had so much anxiety that year with college searching and the workload, however, running took that all away. Running and being outdoors helped me relax and open my mind.

Having just graduated college I still keep up with my running in South Carolina. While now I am my own motivator, my passion for running would probably still be non-existent today unless I signed up for cross-country five years ago.

This was the nature of the school's sports program: try a sport, learn, grow, and get stronger. In addition to the courses we offered, we were charged with educating the whole student. From sports to manners, from academics to expanding one's cultural perspective, from believing in oneself to believing in and supporting others, our hands were full with the responsibility of guiding these girls to see and be the greatness in themselves. When you can see the power that you have—the physical and mental prowess you were likely born with, but your belief in it has been squashed due to various life events and others' perceptions of you—and then you realize that you had it in you the whole time and you just had to coax it out at the right minute in the right situation, you start to believe that you can do anything. And this power is heady. It's dangerous even, especially to folks who had ever told you or hinted that you couldn't do something, that you wouldn't be able to achieve something. Acknowledging and welcoming your self-worth, your own extraordinary power, is incredible. You become unstoppable.

16

Fat Bitch

Americans have a nasty tendency to pathologize fat, fat people, fat things, fat animals. Saying or thinking the word *fat* may conjure up certain images or adjectives:

Slovenly

Lazy

On the couch, remote in hand

On the computer for hours and hours at a time

Big people eating a lot

Headless big people, photos shot from behind

People in those rechargeable electric chairs at Walmart

Unintelligent folks

Fat families waddling together toward some unnamed fast-food source

Honey Boo Boo and her family

Me

I'm fat. I noticed that my legs were big in the third grade, at the ripe old age of eight. I sat on the toilet in our bathroom at our railroad apartment in Brooklyn, probably reading a book from the Sweet Pickles series by Richard Hefter and looking down at my legs and thinking, *Wow, my legs are* big. I know now as an adult that I wasn't fat, but I was definitely growing faster than most kids around me in my class.

The summer between eighth and ninth grades, before I knew that I was a *beautiful work in progress*, I was in a program called Prep for Prep 9. It was and still is a two-year program (in reality it's lifelong, as far as I can tell) that prepares economically disadvantaged urban middle-school students for entry into elite private schools like Phillips Exeter Academy, Choate Rosemary Hall, and St. Andrew's School.

The program was fairly intense, beginning with its difficult application process and essays, entrance exams, a host of interviews, an IQ test, transcripts, and recommendations from teachers. If memory serves me correctly, your school's Prep for Prep liaison had to nominate you, and mine, the Philippa Duke Schuyler Middle School for the Gifted and Talented, had its own liaison. To be nominated and subsequently chosen to participate in this program and then to pass an admission test was doubly honorable.

We had school during the summer, from nine to five with optional athletics in the afternoons (which usually meant that we could utilize the pool and basketball courts at the Trinity School on the Upper West Side). Classes were interesting but difficult. For each discipline we suffered through two-hour-long classes per day. Imagine two hours of English and writing with Ms. Feinberg, two of ancient history and writing with Mr. Khan and Mr. Mahabir, two of math (my favorite)—one for test prep and the other for algebra and geometry—with Ms. I-don't-remember-her-name but she was in the military and she ran class accordingly, and two for science with hours-long labs with Mr. Fernandez, the out-of-the-box-thinking science teacher from the Boogie Down Bronx who encouraged my writing and research on adolescent sexuality in the eighth grade.

We also had seminars on essay writing for independent schools and workshops on financial-aid and private-school applications for our parents. We registered for the SSAT, a standardized exam for entrance into private schools, and had school visits for both students and parents, some with overnight stays. There were parties before school breaks, stern discussions for not working up to one's potential, and threats for expulsion from the program—I only had *two* such interactions. There were teacher-parent meetings, panel discussions about financial aid and dorm life with students and parents who had already gone through the process, and practice admissions interviews.

Prep was the big league, devoid of the petty regular-school childishness and immaturity, right? No, hardly. Enter a short, overly confident boy who somehow had been an extra in some stupid show that nobody ever saw. Yeah, he was smart. But he was also a raging prick.

Even though the program was for high-achieving students, or nerds/geeks as some called us, there was still a pecking order, and I was pretty much at the bottom of it. I was extremely shy and introverted (the two aren't mutually exclusive), which for most people who have only known me in adulthood is probably hard to believe.

I had few friends; in fact, I didn't really have any peers I could call friends who I could hang out with and invite over to our apartment. Read: I had *no* social skills to speak of, even around the multitude of cousins with whom I lived in the same building. My real friends were books and adults. Books didn't care that I could hold an interesting conversation with adults. They also didn't care that I wasn't quick-witted. They *did* care that I knew the entire anatomy of the pancreas and how to pronounce "islets of Langerhans," or that I could quickly find logarithms at the back of my math book (calculators do that now). Books thought I was cool for having read the entirety of the V. C. Andrews *Flowers in the Attic* series in fifth grade and for having already determined that I was going to be a gastroenterologist. Hence, I hung out with them and my journals, scribbling away furiously, especially after bad days at school, and there were many.

Our classes at Prep were held at the Trinity School during the school year. Most of us traveled from the outer boroughs to the block-long campus on West Ninety-First Street. I enjoyed traveling on the subway alone—because this is how city folk do—but I also enjoyed being on the fringes of the packs of popular students, just to observe them and on the off chance that I might actually be included in their antics.

I tried various combinations of subway trains to get to Prep. The most direct way was the L to the 1, 2, or 3. But that was too boring, especially because the boy I had a major crush on sometimes took the J with the popular kids.

One particular day was special. Some bright young minds had decided that it would be National Butt Day. Yes, *National Butt Day*. By the way, there was nothing national about it; in fact, I don't even think it was a state- or city-wide thing, just something that some kids (most likely boys—I know I'm stereotyping here, but I'm pretty sure I know who started this trend, and they weren't girls) came up with.

What did people do during National Butt Day? Did they shake their booties? Twerking wasn't a thing yet, so *no*.

Did they do jump squats and lunges up and down the school hallways? *No*.

Did they do box jumps? *No*, *no*, and *no*.

Essentially, people went around slapping other unsuspecting people on their butts, backsides, booties . . . all day long. Usually this slapping only happened within your social circle, and you didn't dare slap someone's behind in another circle unless you were already cool on a one-to-one basis. Good thing I wasn't part of any social circle. I was usually happy hanging out by myself and with my books.

On this unsuspecting day, I stood on the train, holding on to the sticky pole so I wouldn't fall, rocking back and forth, side to side with the jerky and smooth movements of the train. I was reading. I was always reading. It was probably *The Catcher in the Rye* because I remember being so engrossed by Holden Caulfield's life and troubles that I took no notice of where I actually was and what was going on around me.

Then I heard laughter—a sudden, raucous adolescent laughter that signified someone had done something so funny that it merited an outburst. This laughter was followed by the most painful, stinging, and burning slap to my ass that I had *ever* experienced. Jerry slapped my butt as hard as he possibly could; so much power came from that little body of his. I had been wearing a thin white skirt at the time because it was the end of the summer, which meant there was hardly any barrier between my ass and Jerry's small but somehow powerful hand.

I was stunned; I froze. Of all the times this group could have chosen to include the quiet girl, they chose to include me by humiliation. In fact, I was on good terms with most of the kids in that group on a one-to-one basis. I did (sometimes) have the ability to engage in funny or meaningful conversations with most of them as long as there wasn't a medium-sized group involved.

In addition to being personally invasive, slapping my behind after having mostly shunned me, not acknowledging me on the train, they chose to—or rather, *Jerry* chose to—both include and exclude me in this way.

I reacted quickly and without thinking through the social consequences of my next action. My brain can be slow like that.

Like my mother, I always traveled prepared. In my book bag I had Ziplocs full of baby wipes, granola bars, little pads of paper just in case I had an idea, many pencils and pens of differing colors and sizes and textures, a protractor and compass, and various other school-related sundries. I happened to have a small bottle of lotion in my pocket, the kind you get during a stay in the hospital. I usually carried two or three, both in my book bag and in my pocket, so I was never, um, ashy. Black people can be cruel when one of our own shows symptoms of dry skin.

Anyway, in a desperate attempt to retaliate, I whipped out a bottle of lotion and squeezed as hard as I could, squirting its contents on him. The lotion landed beautifully all over his flattop (I believe these are back in style now).

I was angry. I was so angry that my hands shook and the skin above my right eye started twitching.

Jerry was also angry. I had defiled his perfectly coiffed, coiled, and sheened haircut.

"You fat bitch! What the fuck?"

I just stood there. I had few social skills and even fewer verbal skills to come back with a funny or witty retort. The moment was so awkward and hurtful, like the kind of hurt you imagine when someone kicks you in the stomach and all the air in your body is released and all you feel is raw pain. But what was most hurtful was the fact that none of my other classmates on that train said or did anything. They simply stared. I was heartbroken.

The rest of the train ride was a blur. I don't know if I stayed on the same car as those assholes or if I got off the train at the next available station. I don't even know what happened in school over the next few days. Normally an incident like this would have called for an extended session with my various journals and diaries on my top bunk under covers, waiting for my mom to finish dinner.

But what did that mean in the context of my life? Did that incident shape who I was? Did it shape who I would become? No. However, it definitely informed me on how others saw me, despite the fact that I was smart, a nice person unless you made me angry, and a great older sister (unless you ask my siblings).

And here I am to tell you that as hard as it was to live in a body a lot of people didn't appreciate because it didn't fit into their notion of what an acceptable body was, and as hard as it was to hear someone call me a fat bitch, it didn't ruin my life.

In fact, in addition to being sad, I became angry. And I decided, right then and there, to be whoever I was and not to let some kid (who I thought wasn't even that smart) determine who and what I was. By the way, he was later kicked out of our program.

Surviving middle school today is particularly hard. Living every day in bodies that are constantly changing, without worrying about what other people are thinking and how some treat others based simply on appearance, can be brutal.

My message for anyone who is in middle school or who knows someone in middle school (please share this with them) is simple: Your body, whatever its size, whatever its hair color and hairstyle, however its height, whatever its age, is acceptable. Your body is acceptable just the way you are.

No matter your age, if you're in your forties like me, or ten, fourteen, thirty, or even sixty, your body is a beautiful work in progress.

I tell you my story to say here I am.

I weigh about 240 pounds.

I'm still fat.

But guess what? I played sports throughout high school while being a big girl. I've run since high school as a big girl. I recommitted to running after a health scare as a much bigger woman and then as a less big woman, but I'm still what some folks would call big. And as of the end of 2016, I've run nine marathons and eight ultramarathons longer than 26.2 miles. In fact, my longest ultramarathon was almost sixty-two miles long. So did I let Jerry, a boy who slapped my ass and hurled a hurtful comment at me, determine how I see myself?

Nope.

And here I am.

When people look at me, they don't automatically see a runner. In fact, I don't know what people think about me when I'm in my nonrunning civilian clothes. *Maybe she's a mom. Maybe she works in the home.*

Maybe she works outside the home. Maybe she's not from here. Maybe she needs some new clothes. Maybe she's single.

I don't think they think *Oh, she's a runner.* Or *a person who runs marathons.* Or a person who does any kind of exercise. If they do see me in my running clothes, maybe they think—

What have we got here? That's cute.

But why is she wearing those clothes?

"Why does she have running stickers on her car? Must be used." (Someone actually asked this once.)

I don't let all that get to me.

I like to surprise people. I *delight* in seeing people's looks when I tell them that I just finished a twenty-two-mile run, or I'm limping and stiff because I just finished an ultramarathon. I was offered a wheelchair in the airport once.

Instead of being ashamed of doing what you do or being what you are, I ask two important questions: Why not celebrate it? Why not be proud of the fact that the body you are in can do great things?

———

I wish I had words to describe what I felt when Jerry called me a fat bitch on that crowded J train in eighth grade. I wish I could express how deeply that shit hurt, especially when the adults around me remained silent and allowed this preteen meanness to flow freely, unfettered, and without repercussion. I wondered if people would start to call me a crazy fat bitch, or if people were secretly scared that I would squirt lotion in their hair. I also worried if I would have to endure seeing that asshole's Napoleon face around every corner.

Little boy Jerry had no consequences for his ugly action. He didn't suffer socially, nor did any adult or peer on that train reprimand him. I was sad for a few days afterward, but the incident didn't determine who

I was, nor does anything like that define me today. From time to time, it still remains a discomfiting recollection despite my efforts to erase it from the deep recesses of my subconscious. That said, I am lucky to have had (and today still have) a family and circle of friends that didn't prize a certain physical aesthetic over another. I'm lucky to have been raised in a loving and positive-body-image household. This is my wish for all young people and adults.

———

After a couple of days, the National Butt Day incident stopped permeating my every thought. I continued to give that little boy a nasty look whenever I passed him. He had hurt me, but I kept reminding myself that I was smart, that I had a family who loved me, and that I wasn't a bitch. I was fat, yes, but I wasn't a bitch. I was still someone whom people loved, but most of all, I loved myself wholly and unabashedly. That was all that mattered.

17

PUBERTY, FOOD, AND TROLLS

I had been feeling light-headed and nauseated at school that day in May of 1989. I walked home afterward and went straight to bed, mentioning to my grandmother that I thought I was coming down with the stomach flu. She let me nap as she puttered around the kitchen, preparing dinner for me and my brother Duke.

I awoke to a strange, pulsating pain in my abdomen along with a warm gush. *Oh no,* I thought. *I peed on myself. I'm too old for this. I can't let Grandma know.* I rushed to the bathroom and pulled down my panties to see a large, wet, dark-brown stain.

I think this is my period. I called out, "Grandma, I think I got my, um, period?"

She rushed over to the bathroom and inspected my underwear.

"Oh, Poopsy Woopsy—you a woman now!" she exclaimed, giving me an awkward hug in the bathroom. "Wash your panties out with soap and cold water and hang them up. I'll go get you some clean ones and a maxi pad."

"Ew," I said, wrinkling my brow. "This is nasty." I felt a wave of nausea and promptly vomited all over the bathroom floor.

In the fifth grade, at the age of nine, when I got my first period, I knew everything a nine-year-old could know about periods and Stayfree Maxi pads. I had read extensively about menstruation in the multitude of medical books lying around the apartment.

In addition, my mother was *uncomfortably* open and honest about the normal bodily functions of women and girls. She told no lies and didn't try to pretty it up with any *Oh honey, it's a beautiful process, blah-blah-blah* bullshit.

My Flintstones feet were already a size 10, and finding shoes that were appropriate for a child in that size wasn't easy. We often ended up having to buy shoes at Coward's in downtown Brooklyn.

Coward's was one of those old-fashioned shoe stores on a busy commercial street that felt like it had been in business since shoes were invented. Everyone knew where to go to purchase thick and comfortable shoes to wear for your nursing or teaching job, or for a service at a conservative church or synagogue. All their shoes were incredibly expensive, leather-uppered, and *not. cute. at. all.* But because my feet were so big and they were carrying a big girl, I needed shoes that could stand the beating and would last for at least a year. We ended up choosing dark-blue old-lady pumps with a skinny leather bow. They weren't at all stylish, and the comfort level far surpassed their fashion utility. These thick shoes were to go with my new birthday outfit: white jeans, a red button-down top, and a candy corsage dotted with nine pieces of chewy deliciousness. The night before my ninth birthday my mother straightened my hair with the hot comb, sizzling through the dense coils that covered every inch of my scalp, and set my hair in pink-and-black foam rollers. My hair was long for a black girl. Before I left for school the next day, she combed out the curls until they were just past my shoulder.

I looked hot and felt invincible. Although I had a dimpled baby face, my body resembled that of a young woman. My big-for-a-fifth-grader's body started to garner unwanted attention as it began the process of blossoming into young womanhood. Men looked at me, often following me as I walked up the block and around the corner to school.

That day I walked to school in my new outfit, probably switching my ass because I thought I was grown-up. Before the school day started, the kids played in the school yard until the teacher on yard duty, likely Mr. Halloran, sounded the bullhorn for us to line up by class and then walk in two straight lines up the four flights of stairs to our fifth-grade classrooms.

I arrived at the school yard that always smelled like a pot of boiling pasta as I did every day, about twenty minutes before the bullhorn sounded. I strutted into the yard through the two huge chain-link doors, clacking my old-lady pumps loudly across the asphalt when a few boys from my class started to line up behind me, giving me little nine- and ten-year-old leering looks.

I felt odd in this grown woman's body. I couldn't fit into kids' clothing or shoes anymore. My hips were too wide, my legs too thick. My breasts had started growing rapidly, and I needed a training bra in a bad way. I was living in a body that was more developed than I was emotionally or intellectually. I was on the taller end of the middle-school height spectrum, as I had shot up fairly quickly. I had the physical mannerisms of a young woman, with none of the requisite preteen corporeal awkwardness—I like to tell myself—so people thought I was much older. I could hold lively conversations with adults. I was a reader and a writer. I delighted in doing difficult high school math problems. By the end of fifth grade I had read the entire Baby-Sitters Club series. I read thick tomes like the heavy *AMA Family Medical Guide* and whatever the mid-1980s version was of *The Teenage Body*. I was in the adult class in Sunday school, and I had a fairly annoying penchant for correcting people as they read or talked. "Liberry" was *"library, l-i-b-r-a-r-y,"* I would say in a nasty, know-it-all authoritarian voice. The leader of our church, the avuncular Pastor William Storey, chose me to give an evening Sunday service presentation on diabetes mellitus, complete with a carefully drawn diagram of the pancreas. I was an old soul in an older-than-I-looked body. Even then, I had no problem with my own hips and curves because that's the way most of the people in my family were shaped.

No one had called me fat until that summer after middle school, in 1989. Jerry, or Mr. National Butt Day, and the doctor who performed my yearly physical before I went off to boarding school were the first. I'd never felt any shame about my body, but I did wonder why I was growing so fast. I was also somewhat uncomfortable with all the attention this bigger body garnered from grown men. I was frustrated that the clothes I wanted to wear weren't available for my pubescent body.

The summer before ninth grade, my mother took me to a new doctor at St. Mary's Hospital in Brooklyn. I'm not sure why we hadn't used our local primary-care person, but there we were in some random doctor's office, sitting in a small, cold examination room and waiting for the nurse to bring back my signed health forms for school.

The doctor, a middle-aged man of medium height from Africa with a gold chain around his neck looked at me and said drily, "You're obese. You need to lose weight."

Then he left the room. No discussion. No suggestions. No give-and-take. Nothing. It stung. It was so clinical, so dry yet judgmental and ultimately unhelpful. My mother and I looked at each other, frowned, and shrugged. We walked out of the room, out of the dirty hospital, and hopped on the bus back home.

Good thing I'm black, though. Lest you immediately put this book down, thinking I'm about to delve into some racist rant, hear me out. In many black communities around the world, curvy women are the norm. In fact, we, the BBW (big beautiful women), the women with some ass; the women with curves, bumps, and lumps; the women with shape; the women with breasts; the women with junk in the trunk; the women with thick thighs are the *appreciated* norm, which allows us not only to be happily curvy but also to enjoy a modicum of freedom from societal pressures to be rail thin with bones protruding from beneath our skin. So although, in the moment, I thought the doctor was mean, in the long run his words didn't have the demoralizing effect that they might have had on another young woman. So even if I had been a bit shocked in the moment—I thought the doctor, whatever his name was, didn't have very good manners, and suffered from halitosis—his words didn't change me.

He also didn't know me from any other fat girl on the streets of Brooklyn. He didn't know that I excelled in school or that I was in glee club. He didn't know that I had already decided I was going to be a doctor (and that I would be *way* nicer than he was) and that I was going to find a cure for diabetes and other endocrine illnesses. I could have let those words feel heavy, like a life sentence, sitting on top of me like the elephant on the woman's chest in those COPD commercials, suffocating my very being, but I didn't. Despite his words, I continued to enjoy life throughout my high school years, without much thought toward any particular aesthetic ideal.

Even though many black women enjoy a certain level of comfort in the body-type arena, there is more and more pressure to conform to societal standards of beauty, which necessitate adhering to dominant weight and thinness standards too. Luckily, I haven't really felt any pressure to change my body for aesthetic reasons. (I've certainly heard other people's thoughts that I should look in readers' comments responding to the *Runner's World* "Ultra" profile on me, or on the *NBC Nightly News'* Facebook page after they posted two videos about my running journey.)

Everyone knows what is best for fat people, and everyone thinks they can solve our "problem" with some quick-fix pill diet, or seven-minute workout, or a vile-tasting shake. According to them, clearly all obesity stems from a lack of morality and discipline, and an obsession with food. Once, I was accused of having a food addiction because I had written about loving to cook in a post on my blog. I adore preparing meals for family and friends. And I enjoy eating them without shame and judgment. I have a diverse diet that includes cuisines from all around the world. Do I enjoy the occasional fast-food break? Yes. Do I make healthful meals at home with a variety of fruits and vegetables? Yes. Am I knowledgeable about basic nutrition concepts? Yes. Do I overindulge at times? Absolutely. But despite what many think, I'm not obsessed with food as my body size and shape may suggest. A more important question is, why are people so concerned?

In a video that the CDC released in 2011 titled "The Obesity Epidemic," a group of doctors admit that in addition to making certain personal choices, people are definitely *influenced* and *manipulated* by the availability of low-quality food, the lack of availability of nutritious food in certain types of neighborhoods (low income and/or minority neighborhoods), the disappearance of recess and other physical activity from public schooling, and the inaccessibility of exercise in general in our car-loving, sidewalk-hating, fast-food-worshipping, work-obsessed culture. *Whoa!* Does that mean there is more than personal responsibility at play here in this "epidemic" increase in obesity? Could there be an institutional, governmental, and societal responsibility here as well?

Whose fault is it that Americans and, increasingly, other folks around the world are becoming so fat? Unless we've all collectively and extemporaneously decided to be *slovenly, lazy, dirty, unintelligent, glued to the couch and our televisions, eaters of crap*?

In their 2010 research findings entitled "Morality and Health: News Media Constructions of Overweight and Eating Disorders," Abigail C. Saguy and Kjerstin Gruys from the University of California, Los Angeles, observed that:

> While anorexia and overweight/obesity are both medical
> categories related to body weight and eating, they have
> strikingly different social and moral connotations. In the

contemporary United States, being heavy is seen as the embodiment of gluttony, sloth, and/or stupidity, while slenderness is taken as the embodiment of virtue. A deep-seated cultural belief in self-reliance makes body size—like wealth—especially likely to be regarded as being under personal control and as reflecting one's moral fiber.

We have all made a conscious decision to engage in these behaviors and embody these descriptors, right? We all have control over every single one of our life circumstances, right?

Again, in no way am I purporting the idea that there isn't an element of personal choice. I'm as much a product of this pick-yourself-up-by-your-own-bootstraps society as everyone else. Self-reliance and all that shit. That said, there are definitely *other* factors influencing, creating, and ultimately manipulating our lifestyles.

Drivers will still slow down and ask if I need a ride to the next town when they see me out and about, exercising. "We're going to Clayton if you wanna hop on in" or "Are you okay? Need a ride?" Um, no, I'm exercising. "Um . . . okay." And then they ride off down the hilly mountain road all confused and everything.

But I digress.

So, eh? A confluence of factors, and not the general slovenliness of indolent Americans? In fact, if Americans were as slovenly and lazy as our outward appearances suggested to some, we wouldn't be one of the top-ten wealthiest countries in the world. Why so much hate? And why on earth would people with the responsibility to *do no harm* hurl such vitriol at someone who represents part of what is an extraordinarily complex and intersectional issue (aside from upping Nielsen ratings) for many people in the United States? Why the verbal attacks, posturing, bullying, and shaming? Those techniques don't work for anyone in any situation.

Nota bene: Before you categorize me as a fierce loyalist to any one of the movements, let me enlighten you as to their key differences and similarities. Each mode of thinking and being has its merits, but to subscribe to only one of these movements is to limit yourself to only one way of practicing being human and kind.

In her video posted on Bustle.com, associate fashion and beauty editor and plus-sized body-positive activist Marie Southard Ospina lays down the law defining the idea behind the Body Positive Movement. If we were to break it down to its simplest form, body positivity encompasses the idea that "all bodies are good bodies."

It's that simple. Per Adrianna Sowards, "The body positivity movement strives to create representation for marginalized bodies." What exactly is a marginalized body? It's a body that doesn't conform to, heed to, or acquiesce to socially accepted body criteria and therefore exists outside of the norm, on the margins of what is deemed acceptable.

These bodies typically and traditionally *aren't* represented in mainstream media in positive, life-affirming ways as often as other bodies that do conform or meet a certain body-aesthetic ideal. These bodies include ones like mine—dark-skinned, female, and plus-sized—and other bodies of color, gay bodies, trans bodies, differently abled bodies, and gender-expression-nonconforming bodies. Let it be known widely that inclusion of *all* bodies is important in my own health-and-fitness mission. As someone whose actual job and passion is to be inclusive of all, it would be remiss to omit any body iteration.

Here are a couple movements addressing this concept:

*Health at Every Size: Michelle May, MD, the author of *Eat What You Love, Love What You Eat: How to Break Your Eat-Repent-Repeat Cycle*, says, "We use obesity as a marker of whether someone is practicing a healthy lifestyle, but that is not a way of determining if they are making healthy eating choices, are physically active, or have economic, emotional, and social stability, which is important to longevity." This is partially why the Health at Every Size movement exists.

According to its website, HAES "acknowledges that good health can best be realized independent from considerations of size. It supports people of all sizes in addressing health directly by adopting healthy behaviors." Followers of the HAES movement believe that the American society's (and increasingly other nationalities worldwide) obsession with thinness (and, I argue, the privilege it entails) and all the accouterments that accompany the overwhelming desire to be thin—a lifetime of dieting, nutrition policing, body hatred, disordered eating of all kinds, and body-type bias and discrimination—has caused us to lose "the war on obesity." The movement argues that health and body size aren't mutually exclusive. The key difference from the body-positivity movement here is that HAES focuses on our bodies as being vehicles for health and wellness.

*The Fat Acceptance Movement: Ragen Chastain, blogger and fat activist at *Dances with Fat*, and Marilyn Wann, a fat activist and speaker, are two of the Fat Acceptance Movement's most well-known leaders in both ideology and practice. The notion of fat acceptance is quite simple: there is hardly anything wrong with being fat. The idea here is that you can do whatever you want or need to do in your fat body. Do you want to be an athlete? Pass go. Do you feel the need to dress in beautiful clothing that makes you feel attractive? Please continue. Do you think you have the right to be loved, respected, and included in the human race? Yes. Please proceed.

Even though each one is nuanced differently, the core of these movements is similar: loving the body in any state is necessary for humanity's longevity and, ultimately, survival. We have a right to love our bodies as they are, even if they aren't aesthetically pleasing to others. Where these movements differ is in how self-love, body acceptance, and positive body image are expressed and achieved.

Even though these movements share some of the same goals, they often get mixed up in the confusion of a society that equates fatness with gluttony, indolence, a lack of intelligence (there's even science behind this type of bias), and poor health and fitness.

But who determines health and fitness? For too long, many in the medical field have held human bodies to the standard of the body mass index (BMI). Although this metric can be helpful in determining if someone may be *prone* to a certain weight-related health issue because of his or her individual body ratios, the index is not an accurate measurement of degree of health. At best, it's an eyeball judgment, a calculated guess, an assumption. If you think about it, how could it be otherwise? The simplified algorithm is as follows: weight over height determines one's percentage of body fat, which supposedly determines one's health.

What are we doing as a society when we use this sole metric to determine a person's health? What message are we sending? It is clear to me. Body size, although important in some respects, is the only determining factor in a person's health. If it were only that easy. Look at a person who is fat. What do you know about his or her health, his or her lifestyle? Unless you *know* them, you don't know. You have no clue.

Some folks might look at me and think that I don't do anything that qualifies as exercise. Others have suggested I'm not telling the truth when I say that I run marathons and ultramarathons and that I do Tough Mudders. Many are incredulous because what they imagine a healthy person to look like certainly *isn't* someone like me—that is, fat. The truth is, those people don't know me. They don't know that I run lots of miles a week, or that I weight-train three times a week, or that *I don't run to lose weight.* They don't know the joy and freedom I experience when I move my body like it was meant to move. They don't care about any of that because I should be doing all I do just to lose weight and look like a "real" athlete.

In the end, none of that actually matters. I will keep running and Tough Mudder-ing. I will continue to coach young people and encourage them to be the best athletes they can be despite how others think they should look or be like. I will continue to encourage people of all body types to own their athleticism and badassery, despite hurtful comments from laypeople and doctors. I will continue to preach and live body positivity because at some point we will drown out the trolls with the message that fitness is for all bodies, for all people, and for all hearts.

18

OORAH!

"You should do a marathon," said Katie as we walked out of a boring faculty meeting together in the spring of 2011.

"You think so?" I said, curious as to why she thought my big ass should try for 26.2 miles.

"Well, let's see," she said, counting on her fingers. "You've been running for a while now, and you have several half marathons under your belt. And you like long distance. It's just the next thing. You'll love it. I know you will."

True. I had been looking for the next thing, the next *big* thing, and this whole marathon idea wasn't that crazy. It was just scary. I understood intellectually that a marathon was twice the length of a half marathon, but I couldn't yet wrap my brain around it.

"Hmm. I'm gonna have to think about this."

"What's there to think about? You're ready to start training now. How many halves have you done? A couple, right?" she asked.

"Five, I think," I said, surprising myself. I had done five half marathons?

Well, the last half I had done in Pennsylvania hadn't left me crippled, and by God, I loved doing ten-mile runs on the weekends. They made me feel so good and badass and powerful and worthy and . . . But this would mean that I would have to do way more than ten miles. I knew this. I had seen marathon-training plans and had tried to imagine what it would be like to train for and do a marathon. *All in good time,* I thought. *Maybe one day . . .*

"I'll do it."

"Woo-hoo! Yes!" She gave me a double high five.

Katie knew that I would say yes. It was just a matter of mentioning it and pushing me gently in the direction in which I was already heading. It was clear to everyone in my friend and professional circles that I loved running for the sake of running. *Courir pour courir.* She was the catalyst I was waiting for.

I said yes to Katie before I could change my mind. This, I finally thought, would be another challenge, the challenge I would need to get to the next level of fitness, whatever that was.

"Which one did you have in mind?" I asked, my mind already racing with training ideas.

"Marine Corps in October! I love that marathon. It was my first, and I think you'll love it. The marines are mmm . . . yummy. Oh, and it's just a great first marathon. The support is amazing, like there are spectators *everywhere.*"

At this point, I had stopped losing significant amounts of weight, but I was happy with what I had done to turn around the health-destroying lifestyle I had been living. And I had rediscovered every day I went out for a run the absolute joy it never failed to bring to my life, just as it had at the Masters School.

I had risen to the running occasion so many times (albeit, not always gracefully or without a whole host of residual pain, suffering, and shuffling) with respect to other endeavors—the 5K, the 10K, the oddly numbered races like the 8-miler and 10-miler, and then the half marathon. I could only move up, right? And knowing myself, I realized I would eventually get bored with the half-marathon distance, which doesn't mean it wasn't still difficult for me, but I knew where the pain would begin. I would always be the person in between the slowest runners and the speed walkers. I knew my race would be over in about three hours. Did I really want to do more? Did I want to delve into that part of my psychic and physical being just to see if I could do more? Yes. Hell, yes. What else was there to do? Keep moving and improving.

Many of my nonrunner friends and acquaintances didn't think so, however.

"Don't people, like, drop dead during marathons?"

"You're going to ruin your knees if you haven't already. And your ankles. And your back. And you won't lose any more weight."

"I have a friend who is training for [*insert marathon here*], and she's actually gaining weight. Is that what you want?"

"How are you going to find time to train? Don't you have a family? Don't you work at a boarding school?"

"Aren't you a little big for this? Shouldn't you try to lose a little more weight before you subject your body to this? I mean, this is a big undertaking. It will take over your life."

It'll take over my life? I'm sold. If the thing that takes over my life isn't illness, depression, or something similar, then I'm sold. I'm in. Wholly and completely. When do I start? When do I buy my new shoes? When do I sign up for training plans, and should I get a personal trainer to help me cross-train? How early do I need to get up? After that initial bit of hesitation, I welcomed this challenge.

Katie and I signed up for the Marine Corps Marathon during registration (although it took both of us a number of tries to get through to the server before it sold out). Shit just got real.

———

During one of my first training runs for the full marathon, an 18-miler on the Columbia Trail in High Bridge, New Jersey, I stepped off the side of the trail to collect myself. I was just about nine miles in, at the halfway point, for my run.

What the hell am I thinking trying to run almost twenty fucking miles in this heat? I thought. *Am I nuts? Am I in way over my head?* (Could I actually do this marathon bullshit? I really thought this was bullshit at this moment.) *How the hell are you going to get back to your car?* (I had driven about thirty minutes from where I lived.) *Are you actually going to be able to do this?*

I was beginning to chafe everywhere: under my arms, where my thighs rubbed together, under my bra in the front and back, and between my toes. My brain was simultaneously numb and chafed too. I hadn't yet been aware of the magic of Body Glide, a lube you apply to those chafe-prone moving parts.

I was also tired beyond belief. I hadn't thought to bring more than three gels with me. (These days, I can survive long periods of time without having to ingest gels, but because I was new to these massive distances, I needed that quick burst of energy more frequently than I'd like to admit.) The water in my hydration belt was running low, and I was hungry and dazed. I was probably a scary hot mess too. (I wasn't into selfies yet, and had it been that day, I would've recorded a video about how bad I was feeling, and that simple act might have been the thing to get my ass back on the trail.) And my shoes were the wrong kind. I, like many other runners, had a penchant for buying whatever shoes I could find in my size at Nordstrom Rack or Famous Footwear on sale, regardless of what type of arches I had.

So there I was, nine miles in. I had finished plenty of 9- and 10-milers, half marathons, and even a few 14- and 15-milers. Somehow I was able to get through *those* training runs and races without the looming tower of self-doubt I was experiencing at present. Sure, I had had fleeting moments of fatigue so deep that I would consider turning around and stopping mid-run. But I always soldiered on, and I never, ever regretted having gone out for a run.

This run was way longer than nine miles, or even sixteen. One has to take a big mental leap when moving from sixteen miles (the little leagues) to the big leagues of eighteen-mile runs. Something fantastic happens after you're able to complete eighteen miles. The number changes you somehow. It brings the idea of completing a marathon closer to you, both mentally and physically. Eighteen is only two away from twenty and, shit, if you can do eighteen, then you can do twenty. And if you can do twenty, you can do anything.

I wasn't in this place yet. I couldn't fathom finishing nine more miles. Everything hurt. In addition to the chafing, my feet started to behave as if they had never run before on this trail. My arms and back were sore for the first time. (I had substantially more weight on my body than I do now.) And I was just standing there, completely lost in my quickly darkening thoughts that encircled me like the filth does around that dirty kid in Charlie Brown cartoons. I wanted to lie down at the side of the trail in the poison ivy; I was so done.

However, I didn't have a chance to throw in the towel. I don't really believe in angels and such, but a spirit in the form of an older gentleman ran past me. He then stopped and turned back when he realized that a person was standing, half-hidden behind a tree, at the side of the trail. I can only imagine how I must have looked.

"Hey! Are you okay?" he asked, smiling. His tall and lanky form gave him the impression of a person who had run successfully his entire life.

"Um, I think so," I said. "Just taking a break."

"How much ya doing today?" he asked. I noticed his neon-green vest and snazzy running shoes.

"Eighteen," I said, incredulously. *Did that number just come out of my mouth?*

"Wow! Whatcha training for?" he asked.

"The Marine Corps Marathon." *I just said that out loud. Holy shit, I'm really training for a marathon.*

"That's great! You're gonna *love it*!"

"I bet I am," said that tiny self-doubting voice of mine that loves to present itself at the most inconvenient times. I. Bet. I. Am. But I smiled and said, "I hope so. I'm trying to figure out how I'm going to do nine more miles now."

He smiled his big, radiant, and inviting smile. "You got this far; you can do it again. Take a break. Drink your water. Have a gel. And then get started again. Where's your car?"

"At the trailhead by High Bridge."

"Well, you have to get back to your car, right? *You got this!*"

Who was this overly chipper guy, and why was he trying to convince me of what was obviously impossible? Seriously, had the universe placed him in my path on purpose? Had I been sending signals? Whatever it was, I'm glad our training paths crossed, or I would likely still be standing in that spot, frozen and unable to will myself to just get it done.

"I'm Ralph, by the way, and I've got a group called Ralph's Runners, and we're out here every weekend. I've got my girls doing twenty-two today. They're also doing MCM. Listen, I gotta go, but we have a group on Facebook. I'd love for you to join. Look us up! What's your name by the way?" he asked.

"Mirna."

"Mirna, it was nice to meet you. Remember, you got this far . . ."

"Thanks, Ralph!"

And then off he ran.

Twenty-two miles? I couldn't even wrap my head around eighteen. *Wow.*

I stood for a few moments, digesting what had just transpired in the middle of the woods on a trail that was lined with gnome villages, real human houses, and random people who would emerge from the woods and greet others with "Hey, Joe!" or "Hey, Dave!" I'd find out later that those folks all lived there, off the grid.

I did exactly what Ralph said to do and managed to finish the second half of my run, albeit with tremendous foot pain from plantar fasciitis, back soreness, and brain fatigue.

But I completed it. This was because of two things: I had to (my car was nine miles away), and because this stranger had encouraged me to finish it, even though he didn't *know* me from a poison ivy–covered tree or a sweaty, smelly, menacing-looking bear on the prowl. He was cheering me on, encouraging me, and transferring his energy and positivity to me.

Somehow I found the energy to run and walk back to the trailhead and then to my car. Reaching the end of my run was oddly anticlimactic. I guess I'd already had all the epiphanies I would have that day after meeting Coach Ralph. Finishing that run was simply a matter of finishing. No celebration needed, just a fierce belief in self and the knowledge that no one was going to do it for me.

As is par for the course, the walk from the car to my front door was the most painful thing I had experienced in marathon training thus far (apart from fracturing my ankle earlier that summer at the beginning of training). When I had finished running, I hadn't bothered to stretch because, well, my legs, back, and arms were all frozen, and the thought of forcing them into submission would probably cause more damage than just getting into the damned car and suffering the half-hour drive home. I was thirsty, hungry, and mad that I was in so much pain. I was also elated to have finished the thing I thought I couldn't do. I was feeling quite legit.

"How was your run? How much did you do?" Cito asked after I slowly shuffled across the living room floor. I collapsed stomach-first onto the soft, inviting couch.

"Eighteen miles," I said into a throw pillow, my voice muffled.

"Eight miles?" I didn't know if he hadn't heard me correctly or if he simply didn't believe me.

"No," I said, "*eighteen miles*. Like twenty minus two, sixteen plus two. *One-eight*. Like 30K. *Trente kilomètres.*"

"Wow. You ran the whole time?"

"No, I walked some of it and took a long break at nine miles," I said, annoyed. *Wasn't doing eighteen miles an accomplishment in itself?*

"Wow. That's good," he said, nodding his head as he picked up his car keys and put on his trademark Kangol hat.

And like that our conversation was over, and he was off to socialize with his Burkinabé friends in Brooklyn. I was left to fend for myself with my sore body and a son who was always touchy-feely and hungry. I was hungry too, massively so, but I smelled so bad (and Rashid let me know—he's always been the super-honest type) that I had to get in the shower immediately.

I had taken showers with chafing before, and I thought I *knew* chafing. I had it all figured out. After my first half marathon in Rehoboth Beach, Delaware, and my second in Flushing Meadows, New York, the areas right under and between the boobs definitely burned like holy hell in those postrace showers. I hadn't thought about these experiences so much before embarking upon my 18-miler. That severe chafing only happened in races, I thought. What I hadn't considered was that my training pace was my race pace, so it didn't matter.

In the shower, the burning sensation all over my body was akin to being dipped in a vat of not-quite-quick-acting acid. I felt like I was chafing all over again and for a moment actually considered just smelling bad all day. But then that would mean more insistent prodding from the boy who wasn't afraid to say stuff like "Mom, you really need to take a shower." And "Mom, why do you smell so bad after you run?" And "Mom, aren't you going to take a shower? You just ran."

After that particular sufferfest was over (coupled with the increasing stiffness and soreness from the morning's activities), I struggled to put clothes on that wouldn't irritate, well, my entire body. And then there was the onslaught of needs and wants from the then seven-year-old.

"Mom, I'm hungry."

"Did Daddy not make breakfast?"

"Yes, but I'm still hungry."

"Well, you'll have to wait."

"I can't wait, Mom. I'm a growing boy."

And with that, I was thrown back into the role of Mommy, not that I'd ever left that particular role.

I made the perpetually hungry child some pasta and noshed on quite a bit of it myself.

I'd like to say that I took the most glorious nap ever, but I had papers to grade, a kid to entertain, and tons of other things to do that immediately shook me out of my post-long-run low-blood stupor.

———

Even though sustaining myself throughout the day became a challenge during training, I felt like I was making progress toward getting closer to the top of my physical game, even if I still had a long way to go.

I looked forward to training with my cross-country girls in the afternoons, even on days that were hard and extremely long, like when I was on dorm duty that evening, which entailed supervising study hall; checking girls into the dorm afterward; dealing with roommate squabbles, among other things; and being on call overnight.

Such became the rhythm of my weekends, and most of the time I looked forward to this time, even in the rain. I was preparing to do the hardest thing I had ever done in my life, and most of the time I enjoyed it immensely. I spent all week obsessively devising routes, driving them, imagining how I'd feel at this and that mile, and visualizing how I'd feel after having crushed it. I started connecting two, four, and nine miles to form 16- and 18-milers. I would run two-mile loops around campus if I was on duty. For brunch I'd take a break, do my dorm rounds, and then finish my runs to the amazement of the girls on campus.

"Oh my God, Ms. Valerio, how many loops did you do?" students would ask me.

"Oh, like seven or eight. I stopped counting."

"Well, we counted eight. Wow!"

———

On another eighteen-mile training run on that same Columbia Trail, from a different direction, I hit another wall. This time, though, the wall wasn't due to the overwhelming amount of mileage I had left to run, but the fact that I hadn't eaten breakfast. Normally, I didn't need to eat beforehand, but I had started this run two hours later than usual, taking advantage of a rare chance to sleep in.

I bonked about thirteen miles in, well beyond the nine miles of weeks before. My legs started to feel weak and shaky, and I started to feel nauseated and faint. I knew I was near a road and hoped that there would be somewhere for me to eat, drink, and use the bathroom.

I had seen signs for Bex Eatery, but I had no idea which direction it was in. I stopped a man out on the trail walking his dog and asked if he knew where the nearest store was so I could get a drink and maybe something to eat.

I started walking in the opposite direction in a daze. A turkey club sounded great. Its toasted double-stacked image kept floating around in my head as I made my way across the street, not paying any attention to possible traffic on the road. I looked into all the storefronts: a consignment store, a yarn place, one of those requisite stores that sells everything and nothing, and finally the Bex Eatery. I looked longingly in the window, and like a tourist who has just seen the Saks Fifth Avenue Christmas display for the first time, I gasped.

Here was restoration. Here was assurance that I wouldn't faint on the trail. Hell, I might even make it back to my car. I opened the door and looked at the offerings. I had only brought a ten-dollar bill along on the run, never expecting to use it. The menu had Scotch eggs, three different salads (one with quinoa, and others with a base of mesclun and light vinaigrette). They offered ham and Gruyère melts, muesli, and pastries. I finally settled on what my wallet could do and what I thought would give me enough energy to make it through the final five miles of my run. Homemade apple-cider donut holes with fresh raspberry jam, and some dark and steamy fair-trade coffee. I pumped some vanilla-bean simple syrup into the coffee and then settled my sweaty butt into one of the café's chairs. Yeah, I left a sweaty imprint . . .

I remained in the café the half an hour it took for me to feel replenished. I vowed to visit often and try everything on the menu (which I did—it would become my favorite spot for brunch on the weekends). I used the bathroom, realizing that I was extremely dehydrated, deeply yellow pee and all, and drank two bottles of water before heading back out onto the trail.

That run was one to remember. I'd never been in a physical state in which I felt imperiled, as in, if I were to continue without taking care of the dizziness and shakiness, I probably would have fainted or wandered into some serial murderer's lair in my state of delirium.

———

I ran my first 20-miler a few weeks after Hurricane Irene slammed the Eastern Seaboard. The Charm City 20 Miler was a run that had looked appealing from many angles. In addition to receiving some North Face swag, I'd also be able to visit my Baltimore friends. Furthermore, it was a point-to-point race (which meant that I wouldn't be burdened with the mentally difficult challenge of retracing my steps) that had a net downhill on a mostly shaded rail trail, the Northern Central Railroad (NCR) Trail. *Perfect.*

This race was my first attempt at twenty miles after two rather interesting 18-milers. There would be an aid station with gels, water, and snacks on the course, and I'd be running with other folks so I wouldn't feel so alone.

I had crossed paths with runners and walkers on the NCR, albeit in a car, as I made my way up through northern Baltimore County when I lived in Maryland. I'd always wonder where the trail went (before my second renaissance as a runner and, later, a trail runner).

I looked forward to the event, preparing for it logistically as a person would plan a long, much-anticipated vacation. That summer I had fractured my ankle and missed out on eight weeks of run training. (Okay, I snuck out from time to time those last two weeks to test the ankle on short and light mile-long runs. I actually walked to the woods behind campus and ran the long, straight part of the cross-country trail back and forth—outside of the vigilant and protective eyes of my friends and colleagues.) After finally being able to run during the slow and painful recovery period that left me feeling like maybe I had made the wrong decision by signing up for an entire marathon, I was excited to go and try out my legs with a new group of people. In addition, I'd always felt like I had some unfinished business in Maryland. I hadn't given myself the opportunity to run outside like I had planned to when I had lived there—and my physical and mental health had begun to deteriorate in this state. I was in search of some sort of retribution.

———

The previous weekend, Hurricane Irene wreaked havoc in New Jersey. Although we didn't live along coastal New Jersey, our part of the state often suffered from high winds and frequent blackouts, even in passing thunderstorms. We knew we'd get hit, but the question was how long our power would be out.

The weekend of the hurricane (it would hit us late Saturday evening) I was scheduled to run the Perk Up Half in Pennsburg, Pennsylvania. I was dead set on running it, failing to heed the storm warnings—even the race's organizers had promised not to cancel unless they absolutely had to. I was prepared to run the race and drive back in the storm. I was unreasonable, committed to doing the race, no matter the consequences.

At the last possible minute, the event was canceled and postponed to the following year. I decided to head out for a humid and hilly pre-hurricane fourteen-mile run in our neighborhood before hunkering down with the family (my brother's family was visiting from Arizona) as Irene's destructive forces neared, felling trees and power lines and destroying vital parts of the New Jersey Shore.

After my Perk Up replacement run, Irene came as expected, causing a weird sensation in my ears, making me feel the slightest bit unbalanced. The barometric pressure suddenly fell, and a few minutes later we heard strong winds traveling across the fields and farms. The rain began innocently enough—droplets here and there, and then in fierce gusts that made falling into a deep sleep difficult.

"She's here," I said, with ominous foreboding. As a feral, storm-fearing animal, I instinctively knew when there would be changes in weather patterns, and so I prepared to flee or find a hiding spot until the storm passed.

Camille, my brother's stepdaughter, became nervous. Calming her down and reassuring her that we would be okay took some soothing words and hugs. A few hours later, the lights dimmed and the refrigerator started buzzing a low hum, reducing its energy expenditure.

We cautioned the kids not to sleep by the windows, but given my apartment's layout, there was no hiding because it was all windows on one side, the entire length of the place.

Earlier, we had gathered all the candles we could and purchased enough batteries to get us through the next couple of days without power. We stupidly bought food provisions, but failed to remember that we would actually need a place to keep our perishables cool. About that fish in the freezer . . . well, that smell would go away only with twice-daily scrubbings with lemon juice and baking soda for the next two weeks.

Before we regained power and clean water a week had passed. I visited the gym often, mostly to shower, to give my son an opportunity to get some exercise in the children's area, to charge my electronics, and also to work out the leg cramps that I had begun to experience after having run fourteen miles the previous weekend.

———

My son and I left for Maryland the Friday morning after Irene. The power was still out and all of our preservice faculty meetings had been canceled, which allowed me to get to my friend Margaret's house in daylight.

Baltimore County was far enough inland and protected by the Chesapeake Bay, so the Charm City 20 Miler wouldn't be canceled.

After arriving at Margaret's, we ate an excellent meal of grass-fed beef burgers and homemade peach cobbler and, for the grown-ups, lots of red wine. The next day, I got up at five to prepare for the race. I had learned to lube up by now, and my running apparel was becoming more technical and less rookieish. I ate some toast with peanut butter and honey, and then I was off.

Most point-to-point races have a shuttle from the parking lot to the start line. On the bus, I slept almost the entire time to the Maryland-Pennsylvania border. In between some heavy napping, I chatted with a guy who planned to do the twenty miles in about two hours. He hadn't trained, but he wasn't worried.

"Oh cool," I said. I was hoping to finish in under five hours. We were clearly at very different places in our running.

I finished the race in 5:09 and in pain (mostly from plantar fasciitis), but joyous that I had just completed my first and last 20-miler before Marine Corps. I didn't feel the need to run another 20-miler, because I didn't want to injure or fatigue myself before the marathon. My son and I headed home after a postrace meal at Margaret's.

After a last 18-miler on the Columbia Trail I felt ready, although extremely fatigued, from the long weeks of training on pavement and trail. I had read about people going crazy during the last three training weeks, called "tapering," but I was certain I wouldn't be experiencing that because I was so damned tired. Leading up to the marathon, I could sleep in a bit on the weekends and would only need to do twelve or eight miles. I appreciated the ability to go through a day without shuffling or worrying about whether I'd be able to fit my run in.

I recovered from this last eighteen-mile run and relaxed a bit, enjoying this newfound freedom. However, by the third day I started to get restless. What was I supposed to do with all this extra time? I would still get up at four in the morning and head to the gym to continue strength training and swimming, but then I'd be disappointed that there were fewer and shorter weekday runs to do. I'd run with my cross-country girls, but they were also tapering for their longest run.

I was itchy and fidgety. *Maybe I should invest in new running clothes.* I became obsessed with looking at the Marine Corps Marathon website several times a day, every day. I memorized the course map and tried to determine when and where I would need this gel, those Sports Beans, that electrolyte tablet. I also started making plans for what I would do when I hit the wall—would it be at mile eighteen or twenty? Would I beat the bridge? *Oh my God, am I going to beat the bridge?*

The map showed that the course at mile twenty crossed the Fourteenth Street Bridge over the Potomac between Washington, DC, and Arlington, Virginia, where both the start and finish of the marathon was. This bridge, storied not because it has any historical significance, is the godforsaken place where a runner must be five hours after the enormous, celebratory boom of the howitzer cannon has sounded. If you haven't traversed the bridge, or at least stepped your aching and swollen feet onto its hard-as-a-billion-nails concrete, then you'll suffer from an embarrassment so soul destroying it will (temporarily) take away your will to run. You're herded like reluctant, bleating sheep onto yellow school buses—you know, the rickety kind that smell like high school students after sports, even when brand-new. You stare out the windows, forlorn and envious, spent and sad as the buses continue to trail those who have given up or those who can go on no longer. This image preoccupied my brain three weeks before the event.

The second taper week, I decided I needed new kicks, so I dragged my son to Morristown, New Jersey, to buy a pair of the heavy-duty Asics Gel-Kayano 17 that had saved my arches and heels from certain death only months earlier. I made it a fun trip—I bribed Rashid with the promise of dinner at our favorite Chinese place and a stop at the frozen-yogurt place with all the delicious flavors and gooey toppings. I picked up gels, Sport Beans, Clif Bars, Hammer Nutrition Bars, and other treats I'd later discover I didn't need. I also picked up a bunch of race pamphlets and the thick catalogues that featured the area's races for the next three months. I was already thinking ahead to the next event, which is especially dangerous with your credit card in hand. You can imagine the thoughts that ran through my mind: *That looks like a great recovery race. Oh, I should be recovered by then. I should register now so it doesn't sell out. Is this too close to Marine Corps? Whatever, I'll just see, lemme register.*

The third taper week, as in the week of the marathon, as in seven days before my debut, I was on edge about everything. What was that knee pain? Why was my toe hurting? Do I suddenly have a back issue? Why is my neck stiff? Do I have all the right stuff? Maybe I need new tights. I heard it's going to be cold at the start. Do I need to buy a new jacket? Do I have enough money to go crazy at the Expo? Or should I be conservative and just pick up my packet so I can get the hell out of the Armory and not be tempted by products that promise to make my run the best ever?

This anxiety was so unlike me and how I normally dealt with stress; it surprised me and caused even more anxiety. Other than Katie, who didn't live on campus, I didn't really have anyone else to bounce this energy off to calm me down. No one seemed to understand.

I had reserved a rental car because neither my car nor my husband's was well suited for the trip down south—brakes and alternators and stuff. My car had broken down on the highway the Wednesday before the race, and our truck's brake lights decided to flash intermittently that week, so rental it was.

Renting a car put us behind a few hours, but we still had enough time to eat a quick breakfast and leave before some freak storm, also known as Snowtober, arrived. The heavy amoebic snowflakes began falling innocently and soundlessly against the windshield. The early storm was beautiful, if odd, for right before Halloween. What we hadn't expected, however, was that this light, wintery snow would intensify and become almost blizzard-like twenty minutes into our drive.

There were multiple car accidents due to drivers traveling too fast, drivers who had not taken heed of the warnings, surprised by this freak occurrence and almost crashing into us. A trip that normally would have taken four hours, took more than seven. We arrived at our hotel and checked in. I then made my way to the DC Armory for check-in with just twenty minutes to spare.

Here's my blog post from Marine Corps 2011:

On Sunday, October 30 of 2011, fatgirlrunning became a marathoner.

The morning was a cold one. One of those post-FREAK-blizzard-in-October types of cold mornings. The sky was a clear, chilly morning sky occasionally peppered with flights leaving from Reagan National.

The runners congregated in one of the parking lots of the Pentagon. There were many, many of us, to the tune of about 30,000.

My training had been haphazard due to the painful ankle fracture taking its sweet ole time to heal (more about this in another post), but I managed to push through many a long run, many a missed run (the various maladies of an 8-year-old do not care in the least about whether or not you're supposed to get a 5 miler in that day), and many a day where the shadow of doubt darkened the sky of marathon promise.

But I made it to DC despite both cars having died the previous week. Despite almost missing the last few minutes of packet pickup because a BLIZZARD decided to grace us with its presence in New Jersey and Pennsylvania right as I drove the rental car off the lot. I made it to DC despite not really being able to afford it, but how many people would be disappointed if I hadn't shown up and run?

Of course I couldn't sleep. Of course I woke up every hour on the hour. OMGDIDIOVERSLEEP? C'MON, it's just a marathon . . .

Special K bars and Granola for breakfast. Not really that hungry, but I must eat. I must eat.

Nice helicopters and Ospreys. Nice tandem jumpers. Oh, is that an American flag? Very, very cool.

Wait, I'm still not moving? It's 8:15.

Okay, finally. 8:20 and I'm off!

Mile 1: Nice and easy, despite some hills no one bothered to mention in the literature. WHAT? (Good thing I trained a lot on those. Thank you, rolling hills of central NJ!)

Miles 2 and 3: Really? More hills? Oh yeah, this is the MARINE CORPS Marathon, not the sissy marathon. Nice 5K time.

Miles 4-5: Don't remember: I was trying to take it easy. Trying to take in the scenery, so to speak. There was a river somewhere. Trying to not waste energy. ONLY 21 more to go! Mental games.

10K: Only TWENTY MORE! Oh, and this is not such a bad 10K time considering the last actual 10K . . . well, that was a trail race, hon.

Miles 7-8: Really? More hills? Georgetown. Pretty. Thanks for the Vaseline.

Mile 9: Funny guys with a fake finish line. Fatgirlrunning needed that humor right at that moment.

Miles 10-12: Dammit, where is 13? WHERE IS THIRTEEN POINT ONE?

Half Marathon: Oh, that wasn't so bad. I even beat my last half marathon time. Just think if I didn't actually have to run 13 more miles. This could've been a PR if I hadn't had to save all that energy. Yeah, keep dreaming.

Mile 14: OK, this isn't so bad. I've done 14 before, and frankly this feels better than that 14 miler I did with plantar fasciitis on a trail that seemed to go uphill both ways. Tons better. I got this.

Mile 15: I don't got this. Dammit, I need a gel. Or two. And some beans. And, oooooh, ORANGES!

Miles 16-19: Really don't remember. Wait, yes I do. RUN LIKE HELL. The damned pace car is right there. Scary and stressful. WTF are all these school buses for? OH, stragglers! RUN! Where the hell is this energy coming from? Oh, anger. The legs are like just moving, separate from my brain. Weird.

Mile 20: Is this ever going to end? Here's the wall. This is bad. Yeah, I beat the bridge. But why do I care so much? I wanna stop. This is stupid. That sign that said "This sounded like a good idea three months ago" rings very, very true. MY FEET HURT. Can't, like, jump off the bridge though. That would be sissy-pooh. Yeah, and the girl next to me is cry-ing. At least I'm not crying. At least I didn't stop to stretch and retch. Just make it to mile 21.

Mile 21: Just make it to mile 22. And stop telling us that mile 22 is just around the corner. What corner? I DON'T EVEN SEE A CORNER.

Mile 22: Oh, mile 23 must be right down that street with all the flags. Wait, it's an entire neighborhood? These miles are getting LONGER AND MORE UNBEARABLE. OK, not so unbearable. HI, SON AND HUSBAND!!!!!! Wait for me! Don't move. I'll be back, in like a mile.

Mile 23: Okay red flag to red flag, then you can walk. Purple to purple. Green to green.

Mile 24: HI, SON AND HUSBAND. Meet me at the finish in like half an hour. Where is it? I DON'T KNOW!!!!! FIGURE IT OUT!

Mile 25: Only one more mile to go? This is going to take all day. I could fall asleep right now. While walking. Seriously. Just walk over me. Don't worry, I'll be passed out.

Wait. This is almost over. THIS IS ALMOST OVER? Holy CRAP.

But I don't see the finish. They said it was close. I don't see it.

Oh, there it is.

Another hill. ANOTHER HILL GODDAMMIT!
WTF???? The nerve! Um okay. It's just my feet that
hurt. The legs can do it, right?

Mile 26: A few more steps. Oh no. Tears.

Mile 26.2: High-fiving my new friends, the marines,
getting wrapped in Mylar. Oh yeah, baby.

You can put that medal right here.

19

DABBLING IN ULTRA

Some people think individuals who start off their weekends by queuing up at the start line of a 5K or 10K race are crazy. Other people can't wrap their minds around why someone would want to spend the better part of a morning and afternoon running a marathon. "Didn't that guy Pheidippides drop dead after he finished running to Marathon? And won't that much running ruin your poor ole joints? Huh?"

You can imagine the looks I get when I mention that I like to run ultramarathons.

"What the hell is an ultramarathon?" I am often asked.

"Anything beyond a regular marathon distance," I say, expecting disbelief followed by a stupid comment.

"Well, what's a marathon distance?"

"Twenty-six miles," I say, waiting for it.

"Wait, so like . . ."

Anticipating the rest of the question, I say, "Thirty-one miles, sixty-two . . ."

"Wait, what? You *like* doing that?"

"The only time you'll find me running is if [*insert dumb reason here, like being chased by a bear or the police . . .*]. Seriously, you *like* doing that? Doesn't it hurt? How long does it take you? Why? Just *why?*"

———

As soon as I crossed the finish line of the New Jersey Trail Series Ultra Festival marathon in 2012, Rick McNulty congratulated and knighted me with the heavy, square finisher's medal.

I barely had time to be proud of my accomplishment before he looked me in the eyes and asked, "So you're doing the 50K next year, right?" For Rick and his wife, the codirector of the series, it was just the next logical step. I don't recall exactly how I responded—perhaps I mumbled *Maybe* or *I'll think about it*—but I knew I would at least try. I smiled and chuckled, then exited his embrace quickly so I wouldn't agree to anything else crazy.

The previous year, I had volunteered for a few NJTS events—manning various aid stations, recruiting my son to help make countless peanut-butter-and-jelly sandwiches, helping out with bib pickup, and occasionally driving a runner who DNF'd back to the start line in my warm truck.

I stood by the aid station, bundled up in my thick woolen mittens and hat, scarf, and a fluffy goose-down coat, and watched as runners came and went, grabbing handfuls of candy, salted peanuts, and chips with their clammy hands that had been who knows where. (As a runner, sometimes you overlook basic hygiene to expedite the in-and-out at the aid station. You don't want to linger too long and start conversing—eventually, you'll talk yourself out of moving on.)

The trail marathon had taken me more than seven hours, and I was pretty satisfied with my time. But I had no idea what an extra five miles would mean physically and mentally. After the marathon I was spent, but a few months later, when registration for next year's Ultra Festival went live, I signed up immediately for the 50K distance in 2013.

That mid-March day in New Jersey had meant unpredictable weather: cold, icy, and snowy with an occasional pale ray from the sun. Upon arriving at the start line on race morning, there was a nip in the air that would remain all day (and night for those running both 100K and 100M races).

The trail was deeply rutted, frozen in some places, waterlogged in others, muddy, and uneven. I was wearing many layers (probably too many) so that I wouldn't freeze to death. I wore someone's cell-phone gloves that had been left on my piano at home and my first pair of really expensive trail shoes I had finally purchased after I realized that I preferred trails to roads.

The first ten miles felt good, in a runnerly kind of way. I tried not to think of the entirety of the mileage I had to do. The fact that people on the course would be running all night comforted me. At one point I crossed paths with two guys who complained that they were only at mile forty-five. The word *only* got to me and started picking at me. If these guys are already at forty-five, and I'm at twenty, what am I complaining about? I only have eleven more to go, but eleven was an eternity, considering I would have to do an entire ten-mile loop again.

As in many other events I've done, I knew I would finish (barring injury, but then again, I did run nine miles once on a fractured ankle). The question was when. The moment I did finish was simultaneously anticlimactic and earth-shattering. I had just run and walked thirty-one miles. *Thirty-one miles!* This was new. I had broken some invisible mental and physical barrier. I forgot all my foot pain for a moment and basked in the glory of the finish and the heavy, square medal hanging from my neck. There was no fanfare, and no announcer speaking my name and home state as I crossed the finish line. Where was the finish line, anyway? In the big blue barn. My parents, Rashid, and Nikki were there, shivering in the cold for me. Cito was too impatient to stand around in the country on a chilly, blustery day—and he took pains to ensure that he was *never* in the cold unless he absolutely needed to be. They had waited all day, bundled up and patient, helpful and kind—all to be my crew and witness a race that would change the trajectory of my running life.

One thing about ultrarunning is that you spend hours upon hours on trails with similar-minded folks. Similar in the sense that all the folks on the course have chosen to put themselves through whatever kind of hell they're going through. They've chosen to coexist in nature for the hours it will take them to finish the race, and they want to experience the endorphin-laced high, however short-lived, that brings them.

Running an ultramarathon satisfies a lot of my needs. I'm a social introvert who needs and wants to spend long hours outside by myself (even though there are many folks at a race, I am most often running alone). During these hours I quiet my mind and focus on me and my own footfalls against the trail. I sweat profusely and smell bad. I've even made the mistake of thinking I've inadvertently stepped into dog poop but then discover that it's coming from my cap. I feel most in my element: animalistic, vibrant, and self-sufficient. I welcome the pain of moving beyond where my mind and body feel done. The mental pain is almost more suffocating than the physical.

Ultrarunning is an odyssey, a long journey full of adventure, surprise, and boredom—extreme boredom that will eat away at your psyche until you start hallucinating, and until you begin to wish you could just lie down and rip your brain out and then your lungs—maybe not in that order.

I crave the long hours of solitude and pontificating on the various elements in my life or simply finding the next blaze or course marker. Sometimes even those small things take up a lot of mental space and energy. Looking up to spot a colored rectangle or polka-dot ribbon after you've been hunched over and focused on the uneven trail below you can be mind-boggling.

Is running hard? Sure. For a Rubenesque woman like me, just moving my dense and heavy body across any space takes a lot of energy, which is partially why I enjoy the challenge. I love running like I love playing classical piano. It's difficult, and I'm never going to be any good, even after long hours in the practice room running my fingers through Czerny and Hanon scales.

Practicing more piano doesn't make me a perfect pianist, but it makes me a better human being. It makes me more patient with my own learning and myself. It teaches me that I can experience deep joy simply by doing. Ultrarunning is similar. I'm not good at it. I'm not an elite runner. I'm always at the back, and sometimes I'm last. I don't always make every cutoff, and sometimes I have to be pulled from the course. I'm slower than most power-hikers. People loop me on the course, but aside from some fleeting disappointment, I still want to be out there, in nature. There is still a beauty about simply doing the difficult thing that I will never be good at, for the pure pleasure of having engaged in the process.

———

During the DoubleTap 50K in 2015, and especially through the almost-mile-long Power Line Climb part of it, I wished I could just roll over and fall off the mountain. That option wasn't possible; I had nowhere else to go but up. It was awful, painful, and slow, but finally gratifying.

When I reached the top of that godforsaken hill, I stopped, cursed it one more time, and then smiled. I had just conquered, albeit extremely slowly, what I might have once thought impossible. Also, I didn't have to do that shit again!

Moments—even those hard moments of self-doubt and the questioning of my sanity—keep me going, keep me tinkering the ivories of the trails. Couldn't I be using my time differently? Shouldn't I be deep-cleaning my bathrooms or organizing that huge pile of papers on the kitchen counter? Am I wasting the precious moments of my day?

No, this is where I need to be, and I discover that every time. I need to be here, on the trails, running and hiking for the twelve-plus hours it will take me to finish this or that ultra. Running is a cleansing, life-changing, and deeply fulfilling odyssey that continues to bring me to new heights and new lows. During this journey, I approach the human being that I am meant to be.

20

The High Art of DNFing

A few weeks before the Oconee 50K in May of 2014 in South Carolina, I ran what would be my longest training run on an unseasonably warm day. I ran and walked on our school's cross-country course that offered shaded woods and a beautiful view of the lake. I explored trails I hadn't already covered in cross-country practice. I ran to the Rabun Gap Middle School, up a gently rolling country road that offered magnificent views of horse farms and wide-open fields framed by short hills, over which lay a river and a dirt road to the next town south.

I returned to our campus and hopped in a pool full of colleagues who had waited for me to finish my run so we could all swim together. My muscles relaxed as I settled into my awkward freestyle after having been on the road and trail for more than five hours. My foot pain subsided, and I forgot any soreness that had started to speak for the time being. The water was calming and reassuring. I felt strong and ready for what would be a test of my endurance, the ability to keep going despite hills that to the race director, Sean Blanton, were imperceptible. Yep, that's what he said. *Imperceptible.*

I had completed the New Jersey Trail Series Ultra Festival 50K the year before, so the Oconee 50K would be my second ultra and first race in the South. I had trained for Oconee, finding undulating, serpentine trails to run in northeast Georgia and doing long runs on the weekends. I was excited for the opportunity to prove that I could run in this new environment and in these storied, smoothed-over, and wise peaks that some southern writers referred to as "them thar mountains."

The race was to be held in Oconee State Park, a picturesque combination of mountains, mountain laurel, a rhododendron-choked forest, winding trails, and, in late spring, the smell of wood smoke emanating from campgrounds. It would be an hour's drive from Rabun Gap, in the deep dark of the morning. The night before I would be on dorm duty, and after checking the girls in at 11:15 p.m., I finally headed home to prepare for the race. I fell asleep and startled awake after a few hours. I rushed to dress, inhaled some hot black coffee, and munched on some breakfast biscuits. I left my house feeling groggy but energized and ready for another adventure, what I called "switchbacking," southern-style.

I arrived at the start line and marveled at the folks donned in headlamps and all manner of hydration packs. They milled about, shaking their legs, jumping in place, and rubbing their hands together. Some chatted nervously.

"I don't know what to expect. This is my first ultra," one small woman with blond hair in a tight ponytail said to another woman. "I've never done anything longer than a half."

The other woman reassured her. "Wow. Um . . . It's gonna suck, but you'll be fine."

I listened to this exchange and smiled broadly, inhaling the cold damp air of the Blue Ridge Mountains. I didn't care who saw me. *I'm here. I'm back,* I thought. *This is where I'm meant to be, with my people.*

The race began with two miles through dark forest—my first time running in completely dark woods, but I was only slightly afraid. There was no threat of thunder, and after I realized that the imagined lurking bears would probably have no interest in me, the unease I had at the start of the race disappeared. Of course, it helped that I knew it would be light soon, and that I could at least hear and see other people on the trail in front of me, the light from their headlamps bouncing lightly as they crossed the terrain I would later encounter. I quickly fell to last place, and I was okay with that. No one would hear or see me tripping over what seemed like all of the branches and all of the rocks. No one would see me gasp at my own dark shadow or yelp when I thought an owl was about to swoop down and plant its talons on my shoulders. This was fine.

Despite all of the tripping and almost-face-planting, I was enjoying myself. I felt strong and prepared, and I fell into my easy trail pace. Early on, the trail wasn't too technical, and there were hints of a lighter blue through the trees. The course followed a long arc of a small lake that began to glisten in the brightening morning. The contrasts were strong—the water a deep black, surrounded by the silhouettes of trees in springlike youth, leaves moving gently in the cool morning breeze, all against an increasingly pale-blue sky. The sun eventually peeked its glistening head through the trees, and I was finally able to switch off my headlamp. I became less uneasy and more confident that this was where I was meant to be at that moment, that day.

And it was; I was free. I forgot about the onus of having to coach the distance runners in track at school. I forgot about reading Spanish papers and inputting grades. I forgot that I had had dorm duty the night before and was functioning on little sleep. I even forgot that I was in my annual early-spring teaching funk in which I questioned why I was a teacher, why I did this to myself every year, why I continued to spend inordinate amounts of time with surly teenagers, and why I still subjected myself to the suffocation of boarding-school life. Being on the trail allowed me to clear my mind of these quotidian worries. It was just me and about two hundred other people enjoying a cool frolic in an early-spring forest.

The forest began to present itself in the increasing light, and I turned onto the Old Waterwheel Trail, which would eventually lead to a miles-long stretch on the Foothills Trail, a route that travels around eighty miles from Oconee State Park to Table Rock on the Blue Ridge Escarpment in South Carolina.

I was moving slowly, but I felt good. There were a few switchbacks and some short, steep hills, but my legs kept moving forward. After a few minutes on the Foothills Trail, I heard women's voices. *They must be hikers,* I thought. The sounds of the high-pitched laughing came in and out like a staticky radio station. I was unsure as to whether they were real, but I gave myself the benefit of the doubt and assured myself that there were real people behind me, not hyenas or the humanlike howling monkeys you hear in Costa Rica. Sometimes the sounds would disappear, but as soon as I rounded the sharp curve of a switchback, I heard them again, and eventually they caught up to me. *Damn, I must be really slow today.* As they approached from behind, I glanced back quickly.

"How's your hike today?" I asked.

"We're actually sweeping, and you're right on target!" chirped the one with short, curly brown hair.

"Oh, okay. Well, I'm going to run a little bit now. I'm sure you'll catch up to me. Bye!" I took advantage of this flat section and worked hard to put some distance between us. I needed to be ahead of the sweeps, the volunteers responsible for making sure all runners were on target, tended to if they were injured, and not left behind.

About twenty minutes later, I heard them again after I had slowed down on some hills, this time louder and more insistent. Annoying even. *Why are they talking so fucking loudly on the fucking trail? Can I get some peace, please? Damn. Is that too much to ask?* And just like that—and every other time I've let negative energy take over my thoughts on the trail—I face-planted. At first I tripped, attempting unsuccessfully to steady myself over a few pebble-strewn, root-filled yards and trying doggedly not to fall into the thick poison ivy on either side of the trail. I failed. I ended up on my side and then on my stomach, legs spread (into the poison ivy, of course).

I rested on the ground for a minute. I wasn't hurt. In fact, I was comfortable, if winded from expending so much energy in trying not to fall. I thought about lying there for a few minutes, admiring the trail from my unique vantage point.

A few days later I wrote in a post for TrailandUltrarunning.com:

> I'm on the ground. How the hell did I get here? No, really. I don't remember falling. Did I actually fall? On my side? OUCH!!!! MY ANKLE! Is it broken? Nope. Can I run? Yeah. I'm OK. The sweeps aren't close enough to laugh at me. I'll just lie here a minute. Just a minute. Is that poison ivy? I dunno. Whatever. I should get up. Yeah, I'll get up.

And then I decided I didn't want the sweeps to think I was dead when they eventually came upon me, so I got up slowly, brushed the dirt and pebbles from my knees, and continued, remembering for a brief second that my ankles had in fact made friends with the urushiol leaves. I would be reminded later.

And for the duration of the next five or so miles, they remained on my tail. Sometimes they reminded me that I shouldn't take too long at an aid station.

"Hey, you need to get going, okay? You're doing great!" said curly head. The other woman said little to me. Other times they'd be far enough away that I felt some solitude, albeit rushed.

I came to a long downhill section on a dirt road about four miles from the halfway point. I became worried after I realized I'd have to do it in the other direction. Even the very thin, superfit, elite-looking types looked miserable trudging up the hill, and most of them were walking, hunched over and breathing heavily. I took the opportunity to pick up the pace, even though I knew I'd be destroying my quads.

At a few points on this part of the course, I saw the glowing effervescence of the Blue Ridge Mountains coming to life midmorning, shimmering like a body of water through the thickening foliage against the backdrop of an exquisite, deepening beryl-colored sky. The Blue Ridge Mountains aren't actually blue, but due to a combination of a rain-forest-level moisture traveling up from the Gulf Coast, air pollution, the physics-related light-bouncing-off-dark-objects phenomenon, and hydrocarbon particles being released from the trees and plants, they glow from afar, emanating an almost-azure haze from a distance.

Running the downhill felt easy, liberating almost. I had taken many walking breaks on the constant up-and-downs of the first few miles of the course, so this felt like a gift, even if I had to ignore the struggling faces of the folks traveling back up the hill. It was fairly steep, and I made the rookie error of traveling too fast and hard down a steep descent. All practiced running form flew by the wayside, and I overtaxed my quadriceps, knees, and hamstrings by putting on the brakes every time my feet touched the ground, trying desperately to remain upright. I hadn't remembered that I should lean forward and splay my arms a bit to work with gravity and not against it. I forgot that my heavy body was, well, heavy, and that there would be some payback later on.

The road curved to the right and the course continued onto another trail that ascended for three miles . . . up and up and up, without ceasing. The woman I had overheard earlier that morning talking to the new ultrarunner came down the hill.

"It's three miles of ridiculousness. Good luck," she said, continuing down the hill lightly and effortlessly. The switchbacks began to annoy me, and I became more and more frustrated with myself for not being able to conquer the hills as I had imagined I would with all my training. I had worked on this with hill repeats and wind sprints, strength training, and miles upon miles of running. I wondered out loud why I chose to put myself through this *again*.

After the extraordinary high of kicking it into gear on the long downhill, my left hamstring began to feel tight along with the outside of my left knee as I climbed uphill on the next section. I pressed ahead, stopping every quarter mile or so to stretch my leg and loosen up my hips. I slowed down so much that the petite Japanese woman I had passed on the downhill was gaining on me, and the two sweeps were on my tail again. I couldn't see them, but I heard them.

"So, like, are you guys all set with everything for the wedding?" asked curly head.

"I'm freaking out. Everybody's going fucking crazy, including Ben. He won't even sleep with me, he's so wigged out."

"What's he, like, scared about?"

"I don't know, but it kinda makes me worried. What are we going to do when the shit hits the fan after we're married, just not have sex?"

"Well, maybe you can, like, get some cute lingerie and, like, surprise him this week . . ."

"Hmm . . . I don't know if he'd be up for that. He's kinda like, um, not the type who likes surprises."

And it went on and on. I tried to block out their voices as I progressed forward.

After one too many switchbacks, I heard commotion coming from the midpoint aid station. *Yes. I've made it!* I hadn't been thinking that I wouldn't make the cutoff, because the sweeps would have informed me as such, right? They had kept me moving earlier. I thought I was golden.

I arrived at the aid station, ready to refill my pack and munch on the southern delicacies spread out on the table. Before I could pick up some energy gels to sustain me through the second half of the course, curly head approached me with a look of fake apology on her face.

"I'm sorry, your race is over. We have to pull you off the course. You're a minute over."

I'm not much of a crier. I may become angry and despondent or quiet and taciturn, but I generally don't cry unless I'm having marital issues or a loved one dies.

"What do you mean? For Christ's sake. Jesus!" I yelled. *What the fuck?* I felt the familiar burn of watering eyes and fought to hold my tears back.

"Seriously?" I asked, dumbfounded.

"We're sorry; it's 5:01 and we have to pull you off the course. You're a minute over the cutoff," said curly head again.

"Were you going to fucking tell me?" I mumbled as I stormed off the trail. I looked into the trees and cried. *What the fuck, man? A minute. A whole fucking minute. Fuck you and fuck those stupid, loud-ass dumb girls.*

A minute later they pulled the Japanese woman off the course too. She got even angrier.

"You didn't tell me when you passed me. This is not fair! This fucked up! You should say something to me. I pay a lot of money and drive a long way!" she yelled.

"We have to pull you off the course."

I wiped my tears with the baby wipes I had stashed in my bra and tried to compose myself. I stretched my hamstrings on a nearby boulder and breathed deeply.

It wasn't meant to be, I told myself. *The universe has other plans.*

Okay. This was still screwed up, but it could be a learning experience, and anyway, I was tired as hell.

"Oh well, might as well not perseverate about it," I said to the trees. I think they agreed to my plan.

As I stood by the boulder at the side of the trail, the fact that this experience would make a *great* story either for my blog or for TrailandUltrarunning.com calmed me down a bit. I comforted myself at the prospect of telling this story. I would at least glean some lessons from this failed attempt at my second ultra, and I would be able to share them. Also, I could go home and get some much-needed sleep.

After I regained the equanimity that I had had at the beginning of the race, I turned around and headed toward the table. It boasted a veritable smorgasbord, typical trail-race fare. Both Reiko, the Japanese woman, and I would need a ride back to the start/finish line, but not before noshing on salt-and-vinegar pork rinds, pickle spears, and salty cheddar-bacon-flavored gluten-free goldfish.

Sean's father drove us back to the start.

"So what happened back there?" he asked, as we piled into his cream-colored Suburban.

"We didn't make the cutoff. So here we are. I'm Mirna, by the way."

"Nice to meet you. Not the best circumstances . . . ," he said, a little awkwardly.

"Yeah, I know. I'm over it, though. On to the next one."

"Well, that's a good attitude. My son is tough. He takes these races very seriously."

"We kinda figured that out. But whatever, I'll just try again next year. And I'll wear a watch this time, so I beat the cutoff." I laughed, my sadness and anger ebbing a bit. I wasn't angry at Sean. The sweeps had sparked my frustration and bad mood.

"And what's your name, sweetie?"

"Reiko," she said.

"A-ha. Japanese, right?"

"Yes," she responded curtly.

"Sorry about your race."

"It's okay. Thank you," Reiko said, looking forlornly out the window.

I learned a little bit more about how Sean had started in race directing. I also learned, from just watching and listening to the way his dad talked about him, that Sean's parents were extremely proud of their son and elated to be able to help him fulfill his dream of bringing people back to nature, albeit in a slightly sadistic way.

I decided to take the event as a loss and relaxed into an easy back-and-forth with him and Reiko. I vowed to come back the year after with a vengeance.

DNF. *Did not finish.* For many runners, these three letters are painful reminders that they were unable to complete their task or reach their goal. A DNF can be a source of embarrassment with the distinct message of failure. Unplanned DNFs, as I gather many are, are especially hard to swallow. They remind runners that we are only human, that things don't always go as meticulously planned, despite physical and mental preparation—with aid stations mapped out, nutrition on point, perfectly fitting and functional no-chafing gear, and the right shoes.

Sometimes you pour your everything into one event. You spend an arm and a leg traveling and booking hotel rooms and rental cars (or you don't, dirtbagging it the entire way); you pay an enormous amount for the actual event (but you don't mind, having figured out that trail-race directors do what they do for the experiences they can give to the running community); you make sure you have high-quality gear (and good gear is an expense worth noting); you dive headfirst into an intense training schedule filled with back-to-back long runs, hill repeats, speed intervals on the track, and plyometrics for that still-nonexistent explosive speed everyone says that you'll get. You've managed to expend a lot of energy, time, and money on this race. You're committed and you expect to finish. You've put in the effort, and now it's time for you to shine.

You have high points, truly exhilarating moments on the course. The weather is perfect, or the course isn't as difficult as you had imagined. You're feeling well hydrated and not too full. Your form, although not perfect according to the experts in *Runner's World* or *Trail Runner Magazine*, works for you. You bounce from rock to small boulder like a parkour expert, hop over this and that root, duck under low-lying branches at full speed, splash through calm streams without a second thought, and climb that hill that came out of nowhere with relative ease. You're on the top of the world; there isn't a thought in your mind, except for a growing sense of invincibility. You got this.

But then, that slight tightness in the back of your leg that you attributed to your regular morning fatigue and stiffness begins to speak, and it does so loudly and insistently. Those boulders that were once small and playful are now jagged and threatening; the streams have morphed into class III rapids, and you have no trekking poles. Getting through the rushing water would have been easier, fun even, twenty miles ago, but now it's downright impossible. With the spirit of the intrepid trail runner, you soldier on, albeit more slowly. You remember your mantras, both borrowed and original:

I got this.
I am living the dream.
Step over step.
Relentless forward progress.
They're just miles.
Onward to the next aid station.
This is where I'm supposed to be, right here and
    right now.

But somehow, as often as you say all of these lines in a row over the next mile like a Buddhist monk or a nun silently mouthing incantations, and as much peace and comfort as they can give you in the moment, they somehow fall on deaf forest ears. You become numb and ill at ease. Will you finish? Can you finish?

You have ten, twenty, thirty miles left of the course and your hip begins to hurt too, every time your left foot hits the ground. Then you stop and try to stretch everything out . . . and think, *I'm just tight from overtraining, but I can get through this, right? God, I don't wanna look like a fool. I don't want to feel like one either.*

A potential DNF looms and becomes an unbearable weight that slows you down more, so the pain is radiating now from the entire left side of your body. The once-slightly-imperfect gait is now completely wrong as you place necessary pressure on your feet, legs, and hip just to move forward to the next aid station.

Other runners pass you—some so in their zone that they don't notice you hobbling and wincing with every step. Others slow down just enough to express pity and assure you they'll let the aid-station captain know of your predicament. But you say, still in denial, "Oh, I think I'm okay. I just need to loosen my hip up." Or "As soon as I get to my drop bag, I'll take some ibuprofen. I can make it another few miles. I got this." But despite your valiant efforts to coax your body into submission, it rebels. It is tired. It is broken at this moment.

After you reach the aid station, you realize they've already heard about you. You also know that they'll probably encourage or require you to leave the course, even though you protest. You know you're done.

After a half-hour-long stint in a camp chair, with cold drink and goodies in hand, you acquiesce to the situation. A cheerful volunteer drives you to the start in his air-conditioned car, and after an appropriately motivating there-will-be-more-races conversation, said volunteer drops you off at the finish. You talk to the RD, who expresses sympathy in the form of a cold IPA, a slice of pizza, and an invitation to stick around for a bit to cheer on finishers. Seems a little sadomasochistic, but it's exactly what you need to do to clear your mind of the failure demons. You begin to get out of your head and are now able to express joy for others.

21

FIELD TRIPS

Going on a field trip in elementary school was always a special occasion. After all required permission slips had been handed in and chaperones finally procured, the school bus drivers waited for us as we left our classrooms in neat lines and walked down the front steps of our redbrick, concrete, and plaster public school and into our respective buses. Most of our parents had sent us with either cash or brown bags for lunch. My mother, probably afraid of an impending apocalypse, sent us to school with an entire picnic's worth of items, just so we wouldn't ever feel hungry.

The night before the trip, my mother would cook a veritable feast for me and whichever other kid happened to forget his or her bagged lunch. She'd send me with fried chicken thighs tightly wrapped in aluminum foil or a stack of ham-and-cheese sandwiches on spongy white bread with generous amounts of mayonnaise. My mother also packed numerous pudding or applesauce cups, a Little Debbie cake or two, a bottle of ginger ale, paper plates, napkins, plastic spoons, toilet paper in a Ziploc—just in case—and a couple of Chick-O-Sticks from the corner candy store that also served as a bodega.

The night before, we would lay out my trip outfit, down to the socks and underwear. We then checked the weather to make sure that I didn't need to carry an umbrella or raincoat. I picked out my shoes, either LA Gear kicks or an '80s iteration of Reeboks, and then fell asleep, excited about the next day.

Traveling to a new place, even if it was only a few miles away, was fraught with so much excitement that the night before the field trip would be a sleepless one. What would we see? Who would we meet? Would Luis's mom be annoying like she was the last time? Would I have to share a seat on the bus with that weird kid? Would the popular kids allow me into their world for a little bit and let me sit in the back of the bus with them? Which book would I read on the school bus? And the most important question of all was: Would we have homework?

Our school field trips included visiting places such as Staten Island's Gateway National Recreational Area to talk to scientists doing research on marshes and McCarren Park in Greenpoint for long, humid picnics where we could see the cars whizzing by (or more likely stuck in bumper-to-bumper traffic on the Brooklyn–Queens Expressway). I'd sit on the bedsheet that I'd brought along as a picnic blanket, eat the huge meal that my mother had prepared, and either read a Baby-Sitters Club book or lie down and daydream. I breathed in new smells, like the combination of fresh spring grass, metal from the wrought-iron fences that surrounded the park, and exhaust from the parking lot on the BQE.

We often returned to school right before the school day ended. Some of us would still have a little of our lunches left (I always had plenty!), so we would share and snack on our food, sleepy and contented, until it was time for dismissal.

———

Signing up for and then traveling to a trail race, or even heading to a new trailhead for a weekend's long run, brings back to mind the field trips of my urban youth.

What new things will I see? Who will I meet? Which book will I listen to while struggling on the trail? Will that one annoyingly perky, barefoot-parkour-loving runner be there? Will I have enough energy to blog about it tonight? Do I have a deadline?

I also have new questions: When and how will I face-plant? Which ankle will I roll for the umpteenth time? At which point in the trail will I get lost? How will I find my way back from a wrong turn? And where the hell is the aid station?

I make sure that I've purchased my essentials beforehand: Tailwind or Nuun, jalapeño chips, uncured salami, fresh fruit, ginger candies, and fancy trail mix with cashews and dark chocolate. I follow the weather report obsessively for inclement rain, wind, and sudden temperature drops. Will there be ice? Sideways rain? Slippery trails? Or perhaps just a gorgeous day? I check to make sure that I have enough Body Glide and petroleum jelly to last however many hours I think this particular run will take.

If the start and finish are in the same place, I set up my camp chair and look for a blanket or two to throw on the grass or rocks for after the race, so I can lie down before driving home. I'll even assemble an outfit that I may or may not have the energy to change into afterward. Hell, sometimes I just collapse in the grass or on the dirt sans blanket because I'm that tired and I'm already way dirtier than the ground is.

The evening before a race, sometimes in a hotel room, but often in a tent, I lay out my clothes and gear, carefully and methodically. Waterproof shell: check. Tights: check. Bra: check. Bib and pins: check. Wool socks, and *only* wool socks: check. Electrolyte powder: *major check*. Drop bag: check. Pack: check. Gels, food, and TP in pack: check. Cap: check. Tank: check. Lube: check. Poles: check. Shoes: check.

Mirna Valerio

I take a ritual photo and post it on social media. My adrenaline level rises exponentially. To calm myself, I watch episodes of whatever mindless sitcom is on the one nonfuzzy channel at the cheap hotel, or I breathe deeply in my tent and listen to the patter of feet back and forth to the communal privy, tents being zipped closed, and people moving around in their sleeping bags and on their Therm-a-Rests. I lie down on the overly soft, sunken-in-the-middle hotel bed or my own sleeping pad, but am unable to sleep deeply. I sleep in fits and starts. I toss and turn, excitement and anxiety confusing themselves in my vivid dreams.

I drive to the start of the race at o-dark-thirty the next morning in full race gear, shoes and pack thrown in the back of my mud-stained car, and squint my way through the morning darkness and fog to arrive at the parking lot, where I get on the dark school bus with all the other runners. The bus ride is filled with nervous chatter of new and veteran trail runners and ultrarunners. I imagine the scenery I'll see, the sounds I'll hear, the scents I'll inhale. I want to save every bit of cell-phone battery I can for all the pictures I'll take on my field trip.

After a much-too-bumpy ride on dirt roads in the middle of some national forest or state park, the bus deposits us at the trailhead in the middle of nowhere. The race director will say "Go!" in an almost whisper and start the timer. There is no fanfare, no gun, and then the loosely organized clump of us are off, the slower among us walking the first mile or so to warm up, others at the front zipping off at a faster-than-human pace—our hours-long field trip through fields, forests, ravines, cliffs, and streams.

We'll experience new things, meet new people, trip over branches and rocks or absolutely nothing, reach serious lows, achieve delirious highs, get lost, and find our way back to the trail. We'll cross the finish line elated, sleepy, and hungry. We'll share our beer and food from our personal coolers. And after a while, we'll each get into our cars—creaky, stiff, dirty, and smelly—and head home.

22

DIRT, ROCKS, AND JEWELS

I was desperate to find an ultramarathon to finish out 2013. For symbolic reasons, I wanted it to be in Georgia. I had DNF'd the Oconee 50K earlier that year, and I was still on a mission to baptize my trail running in the south. I wanted to experience the natural beauty of Appalachia on my own terms, by cultivating an intimate relationship with the forest on a most basic level, running and walking for a few hours through the literal ups-and-downs of the mountains and those of my spirit.

The Georgia Jewel 35M, 50M, and 100M races are held primarily on the Pinhoti Trail, one whose blaze is the track mark of the turkeys that roam this part of the Appalachian Mountains just south of Chattanooga. One of the storied long trails in the United States, its southern terminus in Alabama extends 335 miles toward Georgia at its northern tip, where it connects to the Benton MacKaye Trail, which links you to the Appalachian Trail.

The website made the Georgia Jewel look like a peaceful romp through the mountains of northwestern Georgia. Sure, the course would have a few climbs here and there, but the majority of the race would look like a postcard with lush greenery and beautiful vistas from various points on the trail.

My friend Dave had posted on Facebook about attempting his first 100-miler at the Georgia Jewel in 2013. The race had been brutal because the course was fairly technical and hilly in some areas. Succumbing to extreme chafing in the later stages of the race, Dave DNF'd at mile eighty-nine, just eleven miles short of what would have been his most epic finish to date. He had chafed so badly that the burning pain stopped him.

Dave's story scared me. Here was a really fit, extremely outdoorsy guy—I mean, his Facebook name was something akin to the Pileated Woodpecker—and he was an educator at a local adult-education center in the middle of the Smokies in Tennessee. *Tough-spirited, hardy,* and *extremely strong* are the words that come to mind when I think about Dave. I was a mix of emotions when I heard that he hadn't finished: surprised, sad, and disappointed for him. Most ultrarunners put months of effort into a goal race. In this sport, as in any other endurance sport that requires runners to be on the field or course for hours, training requires a lot of time spent pounding the trails, multiple times a week, many at the expense of free time and sanity.

If you were to look at any serious ultra-training plans available both online and in book format, such as Bryon Powell's *Relentless Forward Progress* or Nancy Shura-Dervin's Trail Run Events (formerly UltraLadies), you would notice a stark difference between traditional marathon plans and those training plans that prepare runners for ultra distances from 50K (thirty-one miles) and beyond. For newer marathoners, a few shorter runs during the week, one or two rest days and some cross-training, and one long run on the weekend is sufficient to accrue enough miles on the legs so as not to be taken by complete surprise come race day. Unless you're a seasoned marathoner with a few tough races under your belt looking for the next challenge, you need to increase your training mileage and frequency in order to complete the ultrarunning distance.

An ultramarathoner runs many more miles on the weekend. Sure, the beginning of the plan might call for twelve miles on Saturday and a measly five or six on Sunday, but the mileage will ratchet up fairly quickly, ignoring the 10 percent rule that runners are supposed to abide by. The next few weeks might have you doing a 20-miler on Saturday followed by a 16-miler the next day, the purpose being to prepare you both mentally and physically for having to perform for many hours on extremely tired and possibly already-sore legs.

These plans work, although I rarely follow one to a tee. Back-to-back long runs, those on the trail especially, train your body to persevere through soreness and pain. They make both your joints and mind stronger, and prepare your body for the onslaught of hills, rocks, water, and maybe even some surprise wildlife appearances. Ultrarunners prepare dutifully for their events, so it's doubly frustrating to have trained that long, sometimes running for hours in the dark until the next morning, and then not be able to reach the goal you've worked so hard to achieve.

The mountains of northern Georgia are technically part of the only temperate rain forest in the world, and the rain forest proved itself that day. A hard, warm, pounding rain lasted through much of the day, which is what contributed to Dave's ultimate DNF. In my book, anyone who was able to run eighty-nine miles in the rain on a technical and extremely hilly course didn't fail.

———

In 2014 I was ready to try my feet and feeble mind at the Georgia Jewel 35M course. I knew I'd be running in the pitch-blackness for a while, which scared me to the depths of my, um, depths. I'd be on an unfamiliar trail with hardly anyone I knew. I learned after really studying the elevation charts from the previous year that the course would travel uphill for about three miles, and within those miles would be what the race directors called Rock Garden.

I drove out to Dalton, Georgia, on a sunny Friday afternoon after classes. The drive to Dalton meandered on Route 76 with stunning views of the southern edge of the Appalachian Mountain range. I zipped along on serpentine mountain roads surrounded by thick, lush hillsides, suddenly steep drop-offs, and vineyards lined with neat rows and rows of green and red grapes. The road was winding, and never, ever straightforward, much like the trail upon which I was about to embark. Just as my car had to work those turns, climbing steep ascents and rolling carefully down the equally steep 8 percent grade, its wheels hugging the sharp curves of the road for dear life (well, my dear life), I would have to do much of the same the next day.

After checking in to my hotel, right across from the fragrant O'Charley's, I headed over to a nearby Holiday Inn to pick up my race packet. I was still in my school clothes and probably didn't look like much of a runner, much less someone who could travel thirty-five miles on her own feet in the mountains of northwest Georgia.

After I picked up my race number and swag bag, I headed back to the hotel to prepare for the following day's epic adventure. As I left the packet pickup, I heard someone say, "Wow, she's doing the 35. Wow!"

I didn't know what to expect from the race. I was as excited as I was nervous. I knew I would probably be last, and that I would likely be alone for most of the thirty-five miles. *That* I was prepared for.

I laid out my race kit the night before. This ritual is comforting and necessary. I unpacked every single item and then determined whether I'd use it for the next day's adventures. I admired the black numbers on the coated, waterproof paper. I usually pinned the bib on the right leg of my capris, smack in the middle of my thigh so that I wouldn't hear the paper rustling with every footfall, and also so I wouldn't get a paper cut from my swinging arms (when the bib is attached to my shirt).

I set out my shirt, capris, bra, and socks and then moved to other important stuff: lube, energy gels, Sports Beans, trail mix, jalapeño chips, vitamin I (that's ibuprofen, for the uninitiated), and electrolyte powder or tablets.

I made sure my hydration pack was full of the next day's necessities, and my clothes were laid out in the order in which I would put them on, complete with the arsenal of extras, including Body Glide and Vaseline. I also stashed a goodie or two for when I reached those inevitable low points (candy corn or high-end trail mix). After I finished assembling everything, I snapped the requisite photo and posted it to social media.

After a shower and some fiddling around with my luggage, I convinced myself that it was time to wind down and slip into the too-soft hotel bed, with lights glaring through the supposedly opaque curtains. Sleep and nerves played with me all night. I eventually gave in to their games. I awoke every hour on the hour thinking I'd overslept or that I'd left some essential at home almost three hours away.

The next morning, I woke to the blaring of my cell-phone alarm, the front desk wake-up call, and the room's alarm clock. I jumped out of bed and took care of business in the bathroom. (Pooping is probably *the* most important topic to runners the day of a race. When and what to eat are two critical considerations that may determine whether or not you are successful in a race.)

After a small breakfast of a bagel with butter and weak coffee from the Mr. Coffee on the bathroom sink (ew), I finished dressing after lubing every possible chafeable area. From my toes to my underarms and other unmentionable areas, I applied the lube in thick layers.

I then filled the bladder of my pack with the bottle of spring water I brought along for the occasion, popped in two Nuun electrolyte tablets, and headed out the door to an uncertain but certainly rocky and hilly future.

As I arrived at the area where the race directors and volunteers greet the runners, I looked around and tried to determine if any of my trail friends were around. I knew that Dave, my Pileated Woodpecker friend, who'd volunteered the night before, was already out on the course making a second attempt at his 100-miler. (He would reign victorious this time!) I didn't know anyone else at the event.

The 100-milers had already left for their first fifty miles, and the 50-milers were about to board the bus to take them to their start line. I began to get nervous.

"Ten minutes to the start!" Jeremy, one of the RDs, yelled.

I putzed around, visited the Porta-Potty, and then got right back in line when I was done.

"Five minutes to the start!"

It's always interesting how excited and anxious the RDs and others get as the start time approaches. Jeremy's countdown was full of anxious energy and nerves. Then he ended with an anticlimactic "Go." No exclamation, no gun. Rather, a calm statement that defied any anticipatory adrenaline rush.

And then we were off, out of the parking lot of the Dalton Convention Center. We hung a left at the street and started a mile-long climb up Dug Gap Road. We headed up the hill, some of us walking to warm up and others combining walking and jogging. I started out jogging up that hill, but quickly realized that I would just be wasting energy starting and stopping. I relaxed and took advantage of the company. One woman was from Florida, another couple was from somewhere else in Georgia, and the lone guy at the back was a local. Then there was me, a transplant from New York City via New Jersey and Maryland, trudging along, slowly making my way to the trailhead.

The air was moist, almost oppressively so, but I knew that spending the day among the trees would serve as redemption. There would most certainly be at least a breeze, right? At least to compensate for the pain, suffering, and boredom I would definitely encounter.

First, however, was the darkness. As soon as we got to the trailhead, everyone dispersed, and I took my position, in last place—relieved that I no longer needed to be social, and with a sense of dread. I'd be in the woods for about an hour in the darkness as the caboose.

The trail was deceptively smooth and flat—that is, for about two-tenths of a mile. It turned right onto a steep, switchbacking gravel road that followed a power-line cut. It seemed to go on forever. I was last and in the dark, but it was comforting to hear voices and see bright flashes of light peeking through the trees as others made their way up the first truly difficult part of the course. I continued walking, as there was no point in wasting energy in the first few miles that I would certainly need later on. I had a long day ahead of me.

The trail finally reentered the forest and immediately continued climbing. To add to the ascent, the trail gods had long ago decided to throw in ankle-breaking boulders, rocks, and pebbles. This part of the course was lovingly referred to as the Rock Garden. Its name was an attempt to lessen the mental burden of what was probably the most technical and difficult part of the course. One might conjure up a pristine sylvan scene complete with calming waterfalls, perfectly arranged bunches of wildflowers abounding, hardwoods emanating from key spots in the landscape, and smooth stepping-stones strategically placed for easy footing over the clear, gently rushing stream.

Sure, there was water, and there were stones. Huge ones and little ones, pointy ones and smooth ones that caused the carefully designed lugs and treads on your expensive fail-proof trail shoes to, well, fail. The Rock Garden was an evil garden, I decided early on. But I had to laugh at the ridiculousness. After all, *I* decided to put myself through this. I made this choice, to throw myself at the mercy of the trail gods and goddesses for what would eventually take me more than half a day to complete. The Rock Garden and I would meet again, on the way back down, a good twelve hours later.

I continued climbing up the rocky trail, slowly becoming accustomed to the absolute darkness and quiet (although punctuated by the far-off sounds of the interstate to Chattanooga) and the occasional more-than-rustling of the trees. What I thought would be a terrifying experience became almost soothing. As long as I focused intently on not getting my foot stuck in between rocks, and on completing the first 5.5 miles to the unmanned water-only aid station, I had no fear, until the sun began its long, slow ascent. I began to see more shadows, which put me in a perpetual state of readiness for some animal jumping out at me. That never happened. In fact, I ran across some wild turkeys that blended in perfectly with the leaves, turning brownish. It was especially unnerving that I couldn't really see them in the dim light, but I could hear their rustling a few feet from where I encountered them. There were five birds, and they eyed me suspiciously as they inched forward to check me out.

About eight miles in, I felt two unrecognizable stings—one on the inside of my leg and the other smack in the middle of my right quad—as I hopped over some rocks. I'd encountered my first-ever experience with nature's assholes (a.k.a. yellow jackets or ground bees). The sun hadn't risen completely, so seeing them was difficult because they camouflaged well, blending in perfectly with the dark and light browns of the forest. Later on, I heard that a woman not too far ahead of me had been stung eight times.

I trudged on, figuring out that I had indeed acquired my first bee stings. Would I die? Faint? Need a shot of epinephrine? Would I fall dead right in the middle of this rocky course where no one would find me for at least a few hours? Probably. But I continued anyway, over a gently sloping ridge, where at last I saw the forest as it looked in full daylight.

I wasn't impressed. The Pinhoti is a fairly young trail, still in the process of being designed and built. Even so, it is a well-worn trail over which many heavy-boot-laden feet have traveled. Maybe *not impressed* aren't the words to describe how I felt, but I didn't see the level of stunning beauty I'd seen in other forests. Not yet, anyway.

As I left the ridge, I began to descend rapidly, switchbacking in furious spurts, passing what was probably the most unwieldy and sprawling cairn I had ever laid eyes on, just about a half mile uphill from Snake Creek Gap, the turnaround point for the 35-miler.

The Snake aid station, as it was lovingly referred to, was in a large flat area in a gap, or a valley, the space between two mountains. A volunteer met me at the bottom and helped me take off my hydration pack. After visiting the state-forest-issued privy and bathing my hands in antibacterial gel, I surveyed the table under the tent the volunteers had erected. It was filled with goodies—salty-sweet potato chips, gummy bears, coffee, flat cola, fig bars, M&M's, and black-bean burritos—important provisions for a continued trip of either thirty-three more miles to the fifty-mile point or for a trip back to the start/finish for the 35-miler. I noshed on a potato wedge dipped in salt, a few watermelon cubes also dipped in salt, and a couple of stale chips. My stomach could barely take the food in, but I was well aware that I needed to eat real food to avoid bonking. I still had a ways to go.

I dreaded returning to the switchbacks I had just descended. I'd witnessed other runners power-hiking back up those same snaking hills as I made my way down, and now I would have to do it. I steeled myself for the mile-long climb, but was comforted knowing that I would soon be on the rolling hills of the ridge, enjoying an easier, less technical trail that didn't exhibit anything like a rock garden or the yellow-and-black pests waiting to sting tired and dazed trail runners looking desperately for the next endorphin release.

After descending from the ridge, I entered the Stover Creek area. This portion of trail crossed over the creek several times. It was simultaneously gorgeous and creepy, much like one of those spectacularly colored poisonous caterpillars that you can't take your eyes off.

The valley was lush and quiet; all I could hear were my own clumsy footfalls amplified in this natural theater, the blood coursing through my ears, and my own labored breathing. The leaves on the trees seemed to have stopped rustling, and the loud cracking and crashing of a large branch in the distance transformed me into a feral animal with sharp senses attuned to the rhythms of the forest.

Should I run like hell (whatever "running like hell" meant after almost twenty-one miles) or do I freeze in anticipation of being surrounded by an angry family of black bears? I kept trotting along, like the big horse I am, praying that the huge mammalian family existed only in my head. I glanced to the right with the hope that I would see nothing and then quickly looked over my shoulder to make sure no one or thing was following me.

A few miles later I encountered some men wearing cowboy hats while on horseback, riding hulking brown horses with long manes the color of the blondest blond. Their heads bobbed up and down as they carried the four men on a leisurely weekend ride. They were speaking Spanish. *My people!*

"*¡Muy buenas tardes!* (Good afternoon!)" I said, overly excited to see humans. "*¿Cómo están?* (How're you?)"

"*Buenas tardes. ¿Corre usted en la carrera?* (Good afternoon. Are you running in the race?)"

"*Sí. Y me muero* (Yes, and I'm dying)," I said, while allowing them to pass. "*¡Qué caballos más hermosos! ¡Pasen buen día!* (What beautiful horses! Have a great day!)" Their presence on this otherwise lonely, somewhat desolate stretch of trail was comforting. I wasn't entirely alone. I enjoyed their company, if brief, and appreciated the opportunity to get out of my own head and speak a little Spanish to the folks riding.

Often on long trail runs and hikes, I'm by myself. While I'm at work (and I love my job), I often daydream about being on the trail, alone and in my own thoughts, surrounded by a deep sylvan quiet.

While out on the trail, I enjoy the quiet and alone time, but after a few hours I crave human interaction. A wave from a passing runner, a smile, remarks of "good job," "nice work," or "you got this," or a simple hello with "a great day to be out on the trails" calms and comforts my spirit like nothing else can (except for seeing the finish line in the distance).

And then, after a little more than seven lonely, in-my-head miles, punctuated only by the horsemen and the loud crash ahead of me to the right, I heard the faint sound of music from the DJ (who was just getting started, preparing for the arrival of the 50M runners at the Stover Road aid station). This aid station was the last one staffed by actual people before the final ten miles down the mountain—where the ground bees lay in wait, where the Rock Garden stood, and where the steep switchbacking gravel road was—to the end of the race.

A woman, face and knees bloodied, flew by me as I shuffled along, trying to muster up the last bit of strength I knew I had to have somewhere for the last ten miles. She slowed down just ahead of me and turned around, jogging backward for a bit.

"Keep it up. You're doing great," she said.

"Thanks so much. You must've taken a fall. Was it bad? You all right?"

"I think so. I fell around mile thirty-seven, but I think I'm okay. I'm on track to come in first for the fifty. I gotta go, but if you could call my husband and tell him I've got ten more miles, that would be great."

"Yeah, sure." I extracted my phone from my shoulder strap pocket with some difficulty. My hands were swollen. "Number?"

"Um, um . . ." She struggled for a few seconds to remember.

She yelled it to me while she jogged backward. I was worried she might fall. "I'll try, but there's, like, no service here. He'll be there. Promise!"

"Okay, thanks, love. You got this!"

"You too! Good luck!"

Then she was off, her footfalls sounding as if she were on a crushed-cinder track doing eight-hundred-meter repeats. She was *fast*, and her running seemed effortless. Later on I would find out she was Kandy Ferris, the one who would finish first for both women and men in the 50-miler with a time of 9:04, more than four hours before I finished my own thirty-five miles.

I continued slogging along until the peanut-butter-and-jelly sandwich I had ingested started working its magic on me. The gravel road sloped down gently, which felt good—and I was back in the game again after that lonely-as-fuck stretch through the Stover Creek area.

Sometimes (or all the times when you need one) while on the trail, a bathroom with running water, a privy with a peat-moss pit, or even a disgusting Porto-Potty isn't available. At these times I appreciate my experience outdoors and my absolute lack of inhibition when needing to relieve myself. I've been on enough backpacking trips, hiking excursions, and urban runs to know that when I gotta go, I find somewhere to go quickly and without any embarrassment. Doing so requires skill, a certain intrepidness, and knowledge about leaving no trace. I can't promise that I haven't done what I needed to do quickly without leaving any evidence of my humanity, but I try as much as possible.

So I popped into the woods a little ways off the trail—at this point, I really had no choice—finished up with the TP and biodegradable wipes I had stuffed into my bra for this purpose, hopped back onto the trail, and continued descending Dug Mountain. I knew that the Rock Garden was up ahead in about two miles, and that I would hate the world and myself for the entirety of that section, even the steep downhill switchbacking gravel road. I would only see the light at the end of the tunnel when the power lines appeared, because they signaled that I was near Dug Gap Road.

After unloading, I felt renewed. A new spirit and a certain lightness helped me finish the course, strong albeit slowly. I had lost time on the switchbacks at the turnaround point. Descending on the return through the Rock Garden was even trickier on worn-out legs, which were shaky and a tad unreliable at this juncture in the race. My back was also sore and chafed from both my bra and my hydration pack. I hadn't thought that chafing would be an issue, but alas, I started feeling the burn on my way down. I was grateful that I only had a few more miles to go before finishing and collecting my Georgia Jewel.

When I reached the Rock Garden, I stepped gingerly or forcefully onto the rocks, depending on whether I'd slipped or placed my foot awkwardly upon them. I ran slowly through the hills of the trail before it opened up onto the gravel road.

Even though I don't cry often, tears escaped out of the corners of my eyes by the time I felt the gravel underfoot. I was so exhausted, so in need of finishing, and in so much pain (soreness, normal joint pain that was par for the course). I was spent.

But not spent enough to lie down in the gravel. I kicked it into gear, knowing I would be trashing my quads running the downhills. The trail looked different in the daylight, less spooky and mysterious, and more industrial. I wanted and needed for it to be over. I wanted to glide into the finish to the surprise of whoever had doubted me. I needed to finish because I had to get home to my son and relieve the babysitter. I also had to finish for me. I'd worked hard, logging miles at o-dark-thirty several times a week, following my strength training, and going out for twenty-mile runs in the heat of the Georgia sun.

The last mile and a half was easy. After all the hopping over boulders in the Rock Garden, getting stung by yellow jackets, and surviving that lonely section at Stover Creek, the loud crash in the distance, and the deep darkness of the morning, I cherished the fact that I'd done all that with my own two feet. I smiled as I sailed down Dug Gap Road, now dodging cars that had just come off Interstate 75. I covered those last miles by myself, with my own legs and my own mind keeping me company as they had for almost thirteen and a half hours. That final mile couldn't end quickly enough. I was ready—ready for my sweet-and-painful finish.

I spotted the white tent of the start/finish area and sped up. Where was this coming from? How in the hell did I have it in my legs to actually sprint? Some things you just learn to accept, and you don't question their existence. I accepted the speed and finished the downhill, crossed the street, and sailed into the finish line, a little girl giving me a high five. *"Good job!"* she said.

I came in DFL. Dead Fucking Last. And I didn't care. I finished.

——

Almost a year later, I was sitting at my computer writing blog posts and responding to the enormous amount of messages, e-mails, and Facebook posts and comments about my running life because it had been featured in *Runner's World* that summer, when my trail-running friend Ric, whom I had met at the DoubleTap 50K, messaged me on Facebook and mentioned that he hadn't seen my name on the participant list for the Jewel 2015.

"No GA Jewel?" he asked.

"I didn't sign up—was looking for something easier and then ended up having to work this weekend. Stupid. I know," I responded.

And the following message got to me. Here was his thinly veiled challenge with a slight edge of disappointment. A little bit of enabling, if you will.

"Oh, Mirna. Easy is a matter of context and perspective. You would have really enjoyed the challenge, and the finishers' Jewel."

And then I started to think how I could do it, so that I wouldn't disappoint him.

"I know. There is still a very, very tiny possibility that I might be able to join y'all. Very slight. I'm keeping my fingers crossed!" I messaged Ric.

I searched for all types of excuses. Frankly, I'd had enough last year, and I was *not* keen on running that course again, in the dark, with the whole running with bees and unforgiving rocks again. My sights were set on the Javelina Jundred. I was preparing for *that*.

In my blog I had written:

> *In fact, after completing the 35 Miler with a time of 13 hours and 22 minutes a year ago, I said to myself that I probably would NOT be doing this one again. It was too hard, too rocky, too up and down-y, too scary, too yellow-jackety, too energy sapping, too everything. But I managed to finish, dead last.*

But all Ric had to do was mention context and perspective, and then I knew what he was getting at. Nothing was keeping me from doing this race, except me. I was creating reasons to stay home that weekend and to run the easy run.

And just like that, I was drawn into the vortex of ultrarunning again, through little energy expended on my part. In trail running, as in all epic challenges, sometimes you just acquiesce to someone's carefully constructed and thought-out challenge to you.

Sometimes you need a nudge, or several.

Sometimes it takes a person who believes in you to bring up the subject and *not let you relent* under any circumstances.

But registration is closed and there's no way I can get in, I thought. And before I had an opportunity to voice this thought in writing, Ric chimed in cheerfully.

"The RDs will let you in."

That is how that happened.

I managed to get my dorm duties and trip-chaperoning responsibilities covered. I found a place for my son to stay for the weekend. I rearranged a presentation run-through that I had scheduled for another day.

I got to the hotel late after having dinner with a new fan and friend and wasn't able to settle in and carefully lay out my run kit with precision like I normally did. In fact, I arrived at the hotel in Dalton so late that they called me twice while I was en route to make sure I was still coming.

After checking in, showering, and quickly throwing together my provisions for the next day, I relaxed and slept for the next four hours.

I jolted awake to the loud ringing of the wake-up call that I had scheduled just in case I didn't hear the alarm from the clock in the room, my cell phone, or tablet. I lubed up, threw my clothes on, packed up my room, and headed to the bus just five minutes away. As I stepped out of my car, two other runners eyed me and started talking loudly, so I would hear.

"Hey, I think that lady from *Runner's World* just parked right by us!" said one of them.

I smiled on the inside and outside and immediately relaxed. "Good morning. How are y'all?" I said, waving. *These are my people,* I thought as I stood in the convention center parking lot lit by Christmas and floodlights on the outskirts of the American Carpet Capital at this unspeakable hour in the morning. I thanked Ric silently for bringing me here and wished him well on the hundred-mile journey he had started just an hour before.

This year, the first half of the 35M run had been rerouted for a point-to-point course rather than the mentally difficult out-and-back it had been the previous year. I was elated to hear this. I have an annoying propensity to skip reading about the course before I attempt it, so I never really know what the running will be like until I hear the race director's prerace talk.

We boarded the school bus at 5:30 a.m. and were transported to the Dry Creek horse park to the start line. The forty-five-minute ride there from race headquarters at the Dalton Convention Center was bumpy and dark. We were dropped off in the parking area where several racers had already arrived. We signed in, and got back onto the musty, steamy school bus until it was time for the race briefing, given by Jeremy in a lilting British accent.

After the traditional excitement and anxiety-inducing countdown in five-minute increments, Jeremy began.

"Good morning, everyone. Great day for a run. Rainy but great. I mean, you didn't come here for an easy time, did you? Be careful out there because it's slippery. Please have your headlamps on you at all times. What else? Oh yeah, run up this road and then the next."

The whole group nodded.

"Then take the right fork. Don't take the left one unless you want to run one hundred miles. I think the pink flags and ribbons are there, but if they're not, just keep going straight and follow the trail. You should cross a stream . . . it's only about calf deep this time of year. Go through it. Then go uphill to your right and follow that trail and then the road to Johns Mountain. It's a bitch of a hill. From there, it's pretty straightforward. If you get lost, good luck. Oh, yeah, and don't forget about the Rock Garden. Any questions?"

We were too confused to ask any.

"One minute!" Jeremy yelled.

Everyone was poised to start their watches and GPS tracking apps.

"Three! Two! One . . ." And then the anticlimactic "Go."

The race started promptly at 7:00 a.m. Although I hadn't slept well the night before, I was filled with an energy and enthusiasm I hadn't felt the previous year. Knowing that people were watching me from afar certainly helped. Although I didn't personally know more than a few folks at the race, a bunch of people knew who I was. They congratulated me on the *Runner's World* piece and wished me well as we began yet another tough journey.

Those of us at the back began our customary sanity check.

"Why are we doing this again?" asked a tall guy with a big belly. There always seemed to be an assortment of tall guys with protruding tummies at ultras. Their legs, however, were typically chiseled from all the running they did.

"Because we can," said a woman next to me. "We can."

"Just remember, most people are in bed right now or eating pancakes."

"Mmm! Pancakes. I could use some pancakes right now," I said. "But I guess I can wait a couple of hours . . . like twelve." This elicited some laughter.

"Good luck, everybody. Have a great run!"

I instinctively knew that I would finish. I felt stronger and not as shell-shocked as I had been the year before. I had also trained and raced on enough northern Georgia mountain trails that I knew what to expect, not to mention that I knew the terrain from the previous year. I was acquainted with rhododendron and mountain laurel; I considered our friendship to be of utmost importance. Instead of being spooked out by how dense and claustrophobic they make the southern Appalachians feel, I began to think of them as protective, almost like a blanket. I felt comforted by their variance every time I came around a bend or descended into a dark cove. Their presence was oddly calming.

I had also participated and volunteered for many of Sean Run Bum Blanton's events, a few thinly veiled masochistic romps through revamped trails in remote areas. The terrain had begun to feel like home to me, and I was ready to tackle it, become friends and enemies in the same breath, and let it carry me to another finish.

Because the course had been rerouted, it now started with a fairly flat ("rolling," in trailspeak) section on a wide trail that didn't leave me with the feeling of impending doom and immediate defeat. I ran and walked, chatted with a group of four friends, and enjoyed the flatness. When I say I enjoyed the flatness, I mean I smiled for the first few miles, thanking Jeremy for having mercy on our sleep-deprived souls. The revamped course gave gentle hints about the rest of our trek, but didn't frighten us into submission . . . yet. Those initial three miles were *fantastic.* The group of friends were doing their race Galloway-style—timed intervals of walking and running—so I decided to hang back to avoid annoying them (and vice versa) while catching up and falling back, catching up and falling back.

My thoughts kept me company. I was still on an incredible high from all the events that had occurred that summer of 2015. My running life had been exposed for all to see and hear in both print and digital media, and I was glad for this opportunity to be in the woods, doing what I loved to do and what had inspired people of all walks and runs to lace up and go.

The clear and cold swiftly moving water of the stream at mile four felt good on my feet. I wasn't worried about chafing or blisters, since I had on Swiftwick wool socks and had generously lubed in between my toes before heading out to the event. By this time I had caught up again with the group of four, who had taken off their shoes and socks to wade through the stream. *À chacun son goût* (to each his own!), I thought. I didn't have time for that. I was going for a PR (personal record).

The course began to get serious. There would be no more long expanses of fast-and-flat terrain for the rest of the day. The course offered short reprieves, but they were few and far between. It immediately ascended deep into the forest, snaking up the first mountain of the day (Johns Mountain). Switchbacks of pristine, single-track ridge running and a steeply pitching gravel road led us to the top of the mountain where we would be greeted with music, Porta-Potties, coffee, and chips. Oh, and people. In addition to the caffeinated volunteers at the aid station, we crossed paths with the first 100-milers passing through. All looked to be in good spirits as they approached the first of almost four marathons. Some bounded into the station from the other side of the mountain, looking fresh and dewy. Others made their way gingerly up the hill, persevering and saving their energy for the next seventy-five miles.

"Hey! I know who you are! *Runner's World*–NBC gal! Nice to meet you!" exclaimed one of the volunteers as I crested the hill. "We've been waiting for you. That hill's a bitch, right?"

I smiled, nodding and rolling my eyes.

"I'm Josh, at your service. What do you need?"

"I'm Mirna."

"I know. You're famous now." He chuckled.

I laughed too. "I could really use some chips. And coffee. Do you have coffee? I need some joe."

"Of course we do. Coming right up!"

I downed some black coffee and chewed on chips.

"Sorry we don't have any views for you today. It's too rainy." Josh and the other volunteers were disappointed that we wouldn't be able to see the *incredible* vista from atop the mountain because it had been so overcast and foggy.

"No worries. I'm not here for the views. I'm here to finish."

"Totally get it," said Josh. "Enjoy! And nice to meet you!"

"Same! And thanks to you all for being out here!"

I stored my poles in my pack and started downhill, crossing paths with 100-milers on their way up. Mountains don't usually disappoint. Even though the peak of Johns Mountain was shrouded in fog and clouds, the course offered a somewhat craggy section off the side about a mile downhill where runners could view the gently sloping ridge and valley section of the Cohutta Mountains.

I stopped to admire the picturesque vista complete with leaves just beginning their seasonal change, wisps of clouds and fog that shrouded the low peaks, and a town below.

As I made my way downhill, the Pinhoti became more weathered and well used. Two parallel lines of neatly placed stones lined the trail as it meandered through an open picnic area. Because of the on-and-off heavy rain, the area was devoid of picnickers.

The next unmanned aid station was ahead in about three miles. These tables with coolers and two-gallon jugs of water often stood at quiet trail-and-forest-road intersections. If I didn't already feel like I was on a solo expedition in the Denali wilderness, when I reached the table at the crossroads, the unmannedness of the aid station made me feel like I was all alone and would be for many more days.

The rain pelted the back of my thin neon-green Patagonia shell as I took off my pack and filled the water bladder. When I was done, I looked up at the trail and continued on my way to the next aid station.

I knew that I was "only" four miles away from the halfway point, but what I didn't know was how difficult the ensuing trail, with its multiple ups-and-downs, would be. Every time I thought I was closing in on the aid station on a descending switchback, hearing cars and people on a road below me, the trail would make a sharp turn and start ascending again, throwing me into a deep, wooded silence.

This back-and-forth went on for another fifty minutes or so until I caught glimpses of a white tent through the trees. I could hear the sounds of car tires rolling over the rain-saturated road as I neared the Snake Creek Gap aid station, but I was still far enough away that the bustle coming from below wasn't quite close.

In an effort to improve my uphills, which would thereby positively affect my finishing time, I had brought along my fancy new Black Diamond Distance Z poles. Although it took a while to get used to them while running technical trail, the difference between my first Jewel and this one was astounding. The ascents, while not easier, went by more quickly. I stopped often to lean on the poles while stretching out my back, which bore the brunt of the impact of my heavy body on the rocky, uneven trails.

After a few of these back-saving breaks, I kept moving forward, willing the white tent into my line of vision again. Some minutes later, the road was close enough that I could see the cars whizzing by and hear the voices of the aid-station volunteers.

I spent some time at Snake, knowing exactly what lay ahead. I inhaled precisely one date, three salty chips, and a small handful of peanut M&M's. I had to ascend Mill Creek Mountain on steep switchbacks and pass that sprawling and unwieldy cairn again. At least I was on the second half of the course—halfway there. I left the aid station and remembered that I had packed some of my own trail essentials: jalapeño Kettle chips (for salt and crunch—important after ingesting a series of sweet, gooey energy gels), salami (for protein and salt), and fresh fruit (great for balancing the saltiness of the chips and the salami). I noshed on these goodies as I made my way up the third mountain in this 35-miler.

Around mile nineteen, my quads began to exhibit some fatigue and the first hints of soreness from having carelessly run every downhill. I knew that I had to be more careful as I descended the hills on this part of the course to avoid slowing down anymore.

The trail was exactly as I had remembered from the previous year, although now the ground was completely saturated. I ran the ridge, hiked the short uphills, and took more breaks to stretch my back. I felt alive and in my zone, even if at the back of my mind I dreaded the next part of the course. I came up with a few mantras on this section of trail (Snake Creek Gap to the Stover Creek aid station) to help keep me pressing forward. I knew the stretch would be long and lonely, like it had been the previous year.

I made it through Stover in fairly high spirits, checked in at the aid station, grabbed two gels and some chips, and headed back out. I had around ten miles to go, and I wasn't keen on slowing down. I wanted to finish. I looked at my watch and noted that I was about forty-five minutes ahead of where I had been the previous year, so I set my sights on not losing any more time.

Through a combination of running the downhills and power-hiking, I made it to the unmanned aid station at mile 29.5 and instinctively knew that I would *be* and do better than I had in 2014.

As soon as I made the final left turn onto the trail that took me through the Rock Garden not of Eden, it started to pour again. I was oddly thankful for this downpour, even though I knew it would contribute to some chafing that I would only discover later on in the shower. I stopped and took a picture to commemorate my good mood and the 5.5 miles I had left. I didn't even care that I still had the Rock Garden shit show to complete.

The only thing that helped me get through the Rock Garden was the knowledge that it was the last section of trail, though it took me forever to traverse it. In addition to rocks and boulders and the slippery mess, I also had to contend with several climbs followed by somewhat-treacherous trail. It continued to pour. I wanted only to finish. This rain was no barrier. The strain on my face from the energy I expended belied the inner joy I had from being so close to the finish.

A few 50-milers passed me, and I was happy to share the trail with actual humans. Seeing that others were just as disgruntled, elated, and tired as I was reassuring. We commiserated briefly with each other and then soldiered on in search of the not-too-elusive finish.

After the longest-ever section of technical trail, the power lines appeared like shining beacons in the darkness. They are ugly manifestations of human intelligence and presence, not to mention they also reminded me of that infamous climb at DoubleTap. But I had never been so happy to see them. They signified that I had less than three miles to go until I reached the Dalton Convention Center.

This part of the course was all downhill and not comfortably so. The gravel road curved sharply and steeply for approximately a half mile. It then opened onto Dug Gap Road. I finally found myself 1.5 miles from where I would make a right into the center's parking lot, now lit by a combination of waning daylight and Christmas lights.

I decided to book down the hill so that I could best my previous time. I threw caution to the wet wind and flew down, jumping over a large skunk carcass on the side of the road. I slowed down only to pull up my capris; they hadn't adjusted to my new pace and the bouncing and jiggling it had created.

Every few steps I checked my phone clock. Plenty of time for me to PR.

As I got closer to the end, I saw a figure in the distance. It was the woman who had passed me about four hours into the race, shuffling just ahead of me. She was the perfect incentive to run as fast as I could.

I did just that, summoning up every ounce of reserve energy in the tank, every last bit of gel and chip.

"Way to finish strong!" I said, sailing past her and down the finish chute.

Not last.

23

@THEMIRNAVATOR'S JAVELINA JURRAH

Defying limitations, real or imposed, is at the root of who we are and can be as human beings, and your journey is such a wonderful example. The fact that you do ultradistance races in particular intrigues me—as an often injured, older runner, I so want to train for an ultra one day, but I get sidetracked by fears—what if I can't? What if I get hurt? All those voices that you need to quiet before you can accomplish something great. You've done that, and it's an example people can learn from.

—Clare Duffy, producer of NBC Nightly News

As I entered Javelina Jeadquarters at the end of my third loop, I knew that I had reached a major milestone in the race, in my running, and in my life. I had run and walked more than forty-five miles in the desert. I had survived a vicious cactus attack. I had persevered through self-doubt and others' incredulity. I had fought through extreme fatigue and nausea, pain (both physical and mental), and bouts of insanity and hallucination. I had also experienced elation brought on by those ephemeral endorphins, moments of extraordinary clarity, and long periods of self-belief. The balance of these emotions allowed me to continue to push myself forward; they provided fodder for the mind and spirit, and energy for the body.

I hadn't been able to find Good Samaritan Ray's drop bag at Jackass Junction, but I happened to run into him at Jeadquarters. I handed over the flashlight he had lent me at the beginning of what could have been a disastrous and demoralizing third loop and thanked him profusely for his generosity.

Strings of lights hung everywhere, sparkling against the clear desert sky. The atmosphere was simultaneously festive and mellow, and boy, was I sleepy. I knew that by finishing the third loop I was on my way to the finish, even though I still had an entire loop to complete.

I looked around as I entered the chute and made my way toward my camp chair. It had gotten quite chilly, and I had no blanket to warm up a bit before I went out for my last loop. As a result, I couldn't spend any more time than was necessary changing into a long-sleeved tech shirt, my last pair of clean Swiftwick socks, and my Altra Olympus trail shoes that would allow my swollen feet some relative comfort and space for the last romp through the desert.

People covered in blankets were taking naps on the cold ground. Various crews were walking about asking their runners what they needed, shuttling food, electrolyte drinks, and Mountain Dew back and forth from the aid station; changing socks; and massaging gnarly, cracked, and blistered feet. Some were being given pep talks, and others were being spoken to in calm, firm but urgent tones: "You have to eat and you have to drink. You're not leaving here until you do!" or "You've got three more loops to go! You've come this far. No quitting now. You're not hurt, and you're not bleeding, and you're certainly not dying. So let's go. Up, soldier!"

I plopped down in my camp chair and pondered life for a few seconds. My new friend Adrian had left to pace a friend through her last few loops, so I was alone with my own thoughts. *I will finish this. It won't be easy, but dammit, I will finish.*

I crunched on my jalapeño chips, refilled my bladder with water and caffeinated Tailwind powder, did a few back stretches, replaced my dead portable charger with a fully charged one, and set off for my last loop. Barring crashing into a saguaro, or my headlamp going out again, I was ready.

It was dark, and many people who had been going my pace earlier had dropped out for various reasons. I knew I would be alone for a while, but this time I hoped I wouldn't be hallucinating and imagining that a community of growling pigs was lying in wait. I imagined what new experiences awaited on this final loop. I was now in unknown territory—I was at forty-five miles, the longest distance I had ever run and walked. I decided to welcome whatever came my way with an open heart.

I knew it would be a slog, akin to the last half of the previous loop. Only, the thought of a fifteen-mile-slog looming before me was less daunting than thirty-one more miles like it had been earlier in the day. I had already proved to myself that I could run and walk more than forty-five miles in the desert, so what was a few more? Somehow, in that moment, I didn't feel tired, although I *knew* I was exhausted beyond belief. From somewhere deep down, my mind decided to push my body forward and finish. This would be my celebratory loop.

I set out on my final lap around the McDowell Mountains and fell immediately into pitch-dark blackness. I wasn't worried, though, because my headlamp batteries were refreshed and I carried an extra set in my pack. I walked a lot of this loop, until the last five miles, when the sun's rays revived me as they peeked through the mountains, guiding me home.

I trudged slowly to the first aid station.

"Hi," I said, lacking the enthusiasm I'd had earlier on in the race.

"What can I get you?" a curvy blond woman in a Nano Puff jacket asked. *They wear puffy jackets in Arizona? Oh yeah, it's cold as hell,* I thought.

"Ginger, please? Chips too."

"Here you are," she said. "I've been watching you. You don't stop, do you? You're great! You've only got a half marathon to go. You got this, girl. I believe in you. Believe in yourself. I'll be out there next year with you, sister!"

My eyes began to water. "Thank you." My voiced cracked a bit. "Thank you for being out here."

I continued for another 5.5 miles to Jackass, which was hard, but I was determined to finish; there was no doubt in my mind. At the aid station, I emptied out my drop bag and stuffed my pack with the items I could ostensibly still use—more chips, ginger chews, lip balm, and extra batteries—and threw out the rest. I used the disgusting Porta-Potty for one last time, and then sat down and warmed up by the fire. I wasn't moving until I was sufficiently hydrated, nourished (with more broth and ramen), and warm.

Jake, the same volunteer who had taken care of me on my third loop, came over to the fire and sat down.

"Welcome back! How you doin'? You're looking good out there. Just about eight more miles and you're done. Can you believe it?"

In typical low-blood-sugar fashion, I struggled to be positive. "I'll believe it when I see the finish."

A good aid-station volunteer knows exactly what a runner needs—typically he or she can tell from the conversation. *Is she slurring her words? Angry? Having trouble keeping her eyes open?*

"Have you eaten *anything* since Jeadquarters?"

"No," I said, ashamed. "I couldn't stomach anything, and I threw up out there and nothing came out. It was just dry heaves."

"What's your name again?" he asked.

"Mirna."

"Mirna, you have to force yourself to eat. You know this, right? I'm going to get some ramen and broth, and then you're going to eat. Okay?"

"Okay." I nodded sheepishly.

"Put your feet up now because as soon as you're finished, you're outta here. Got it?"

I nodded my head, obeying Jake. I had no choice. I had to eat. It would help me finish. It might also prevent more hallucinations.

I sipped and slurped the ramen, finishing it quickly. I stuffed some ginger in my pack and grabbed a cup of lukewarm coffee off the table. It was gross, but I needed the caffeine. I put my pack back on, and right before leaving the aid station, I made a video and posted it on Facebook. Seeing me in the darkness was impossible, but you could see the CamelBak insignia from my pack and an occasional glimpse of my eyes in the darkness.

> *Hey, everybody! It's Mirna . . . Um, it's like, something in the morning. I just left the halfway aid station, which is called Jackass Junction, for the LAST TIME. I had my coffee, I got my bladder filled up. Um, got something to eat, and I'm ready to end this . . . now. Um, I hope everyone's having a good morning. Love you all and thank you all for your support. Bye!*

I left the aid station, but not before thanking Jake and the other volunteers who were still acting as though it wasn't so early in the morning. Some were still dancing next to the medical tent, their dark silhouettes growing fainter as I continued down the trail.

This was my Stover again, the interminable section of the course that ate away at my sanity. There is nothing but desert, stately but scary saguaros, and views of the McDowell Mountains, in the daytime at least. At night there was only the shroud of darkness and pitch-black shadows looming in the distance.

A few hours after leaving Jackass, I reached the part of the course from which I could see faint light coming from Javelina Jeadquarters. The sun had also started to slowly brighten the sky, casting a low, pale glow at the horizon. My mood instantly brightened and I smiled a full, face-rejuvenating smile. I wasn't there yet, but the promise of finishing was right under my nose. I could taste the metal of the buckle I would receive when I crossed the timing mat for the last time. I imagined the scene at the end when I stumbled in from running the last third of a mile at a clip that I couldn't have imagined when I had started on this sixty-two-mile journey. I'd forget all my pain and fatigue and would just run, uninhibited by the prospect of many more miles, intoxicated with the joy of taking the last few steps. I'd forget that I had just experienced the entirety of the spectrum of human emotion or that I had felt again, in both a visceral and spiritual way, what it was to be intrinsically human on this magnificent earth.

The sun came up as I continued to move in a slow and painful but relentless forward shuffle. My feet ached. My eyes hurt. My back was sore. Every step was a struggle that took a gargantuan effort. I reached the last aid station, where I emptied my pack of supplies I no longer needed for the remainder of my race. Jeadquarters loomed just about two miles ahead. I heard the beats of music serenading finishers and pumping up those who had more loops to go. I heard the screams of joy. I envisioned myself there.

I stopped by a trail sign on which someone had written ".8" in one direction next to "PEMBERTON TRAIL." The other direction, equaling 14.6 more miles, was one that I would happily not be going in. I had less than a mile to go. I took a picture of the sign and posted it on Facebook. I instantly started receiving encouraging messages and texts. *"You got this!" "I'm crying tears of joy!" "Don't stop now!" "Dig deep!" "Amazing!" "Next stop, finish line!"*

A tear traveled down my face. I was in so much pain. I was so tired that keeping my eyes open was nearly impossible. But my community, my tribe . . . they were all rooting for me from afar. Their supportive vibe embraced me fully, and then carried me closer to the finish line.

A third of a mile from Jeadquarters, I began to see more people, those waiting on their runners, and those offering free high fives and last-minute inspiration to whoever approached. My spirits were buoyed. My step was light, my heart full.

Step over step. Do the work. Get it done, Mirna. Just get it done.
I am living the dream. I am finishing. I am finished.

On Facebook I posted:

> *It'll be a long time before I can stop thinking about running/ hiking/crawling/running while sleeping at the #javelinajundred, #jj100. What an experience and what continuous proof that the trail and ultra running community is one of the world's finest. I cannot even process the experience now, but all I have to say is WOW with my mouth agape. The desert is an incredible place with blazing heat and then an hour later it's FREEZING. The sunrises and sunsets are . . . there aren't even words to describe them now. I had to stop myself from taking pictures! My first two loops were amazing, and I've NEVER felt that good after 50K! I thought, I GOT THIS! And then two or so miles into the third loop I thought, I DON'T GOT THIS. It was really hard until my friends up at Jackass Junction took care of the huge BONK and made sure I continued on the journey. Fourth loop was a death slog from Jeadquarters to Jackass, and then less of a death slog until the last 2 miles. They may have been the hardest. And then I met new friends who saw that I didn't have a crew and immediately became mine, no questions asked. Trail runners*

take care of each other, and although I already knew this, I relearned this yesterday and today. I cannot wait to write about this experience in DEPTH! I'm feeling the love from everybody who sent me messages, texts, who prayed and/or sent positive vibes through the universe. I am so grateful and honored to be the recipient of such love.

24

Leaning into the Discomfort

We have a saying in the world of education, more specifically in the area of diversity, inclusion, and equity. It's an axiom to live by. With it, we will be able to weather many things—inconveniences, moments of shame, those times when we make huge mistakes, when we drop the ball, when our kids embarrass us (or we them), when some occurrence forces us far from our own personal boxes of emotional comfort and safety.

Lean into the discomfort.

To my diversity brain, the phrase means to embrace what is difficult so that you may progress. Welcome what makes you frightened and what makes your heart rate rise. Greet that sense of uncertainty into your life so that you may explore yourself more deeply.

Lean into the discomfort.

To my long-distance runner's ears, this axiom means *embrace the suck.* A lot of long-distance running sucks. But what sustains runners are those moments of beauty, those instances where you feel weightless and unencumbered. We embrace the suck so that we can fully embrace what doesn't suck, to fully receive it.

Some days I feel like sleeping in and reading the latest contemporary literary fiction book screaming at me from my nightstand. Other times I just want to sit on my couch in my sweats and T-shirt with the Food Network on in the background, drink cup after cup of steaming black coffee, and tackle a couple of puzzles in the newest compilation of Will Shortz crosswords.

But when I have a goal race or other event like the Tough Mudder coming up, I know that I can't afford that luxury . . . that is, not yet.

I have to put the work in, even when I know that a lot of it will probably be mentally and physically difficult. That first 18-miler on the Columbia Trail in High Bridge, New Jersey, was exactly that. I was excited to tackle this extremely long distance, to see what my body could do after months of training, but I was also filled with an intense dread. I didn't really know if I would be able to finish or if I would eventually talk myself into cutting the run short. I didn't quit midrun, and because of this, I was closer to achieving my goal.

Except for fleeing my dorm room for the comfort of a friend during a thunderstorm, I had never actually run away from something I feared or questioned. I embraced it, with all the nausea, the slight trembling of my limbs, and my heart visibly in my throat. I did things despite sometimes knowing I wouldn't succeed. I accomplished goals and surprised myself. I jumped into crevasses and trusted my training, my preparation, and my willingness to adventure beyond where I had gone before.

So why run long distance?

Long distance trains my brain and body in myriad ways.

With a focus on long distance, my body has strengthened—my calf muscles have become harder and more sinewy, my quads and hammies more noticeable. My resting heart rate has traveled well below what it should be for someone my size. My big, square Flintstones feet, instead of being bloated and swollen, what I perceived as an ugly nuisance, have become the bony and muscular supports of my big, increasingly capable body.

This type of running teaches you to focus intently on one thing at a time. It trains you to be meditative, to empty your head of thoughts. It creates mental fortitude where there was none, teaching you that physical endurance is intimately connected to mental endurance.

What used to be my penchant for walking aimlessly and pleasurably among the streets of Manhattan for hours and hours, peeking into sex-toy shops of the West Village, leafing through used books at the Strand and the now-nonexistent Coliseum Books, listening to music through dirty headphones at Tower Records and HMV on the Upper West Side, and then finally settling into a cozy restaurant with my Sunday *New York Times* was the precursor to my love of being out on the pavement or trail for hours on end. Something still can be said about being on my feet for hours—even when they hurt from having carried my heavy mass throughout the day—to pursue solitude while surrounded by the hustle and bustle of a big city, the surprising beauty of unexpected moments, epiphanies that pepper my quieted and energized mind.

Tackling a challenge head-on, embracing the suck, or leaning into the discomfort helps you grow in so many ways. I always joke (quietly and mostly to myself or on my blog) about boring work meetings that go on and on and on . . . while coworkers are indulging in hearing themselves talk, unaware of their bored audience. I joke that being an ultrarunner helps me to get through those moments with self-aggrandizing people. I'm annoyed at first, dreading the hour or so that I'll have to spend "listening" and looking alive, but then I remember I have done this before. I have dealt with crushing boredom and annoyance many times—all in the name of endurance, strength, and the ability to withstand my challenges and the discomfort of being, well, uncomfortable.

What would ultrarunner Mirna do? She would call up one of the many playlists in her mind. She'd hum quietly, subvocalizing the words to whatever operatic aria or Luther Vandross song are swirling about in her mind. She'd check off mental to-do lists, plan classes, brainstorm new initiatives, write blog posts. The meeting will be painful, but the reward? The reward is simply having done it, having withstood it. It makes you stronger and more able to withstand other challenges.

Lean into the discomfort.

Stand at the ledge, lean over, and then let yourself fall.

I leaned on that ledge one weekend in May of 2016. I spent a day at my first Tough Mudder event, climbing up things, jumping off ledges, trying to hoist my heavy body up ropes, sometimes with success and other times falling (thudding, really) in frustration, entering dark and smoky openings, crawling, getting dirty and scratched up and quite sore—all with hefty doses of ibuprofen and Neosporin at the drowsy end of the day. The towels at the hotel were all sullied and gross after I had taken two long and steamy showers to rid myself of the dirt, grime, and grit.

But I loved every single moment of it, even when I was a bit nause-ated by fear. Each time I enter an event in which I don't have any idea what the outcome will be, I become nervous. My entire body becomes flush, and I feel light-headed. My limbs start shaking, imperceptibly to most, unless they're looking.

I turn inward and become laser-focused, methodical in my think-ing, because that's the only thing I can control. I can't control my emotions, though. No amount of intellectualizing, rationalizing, and believing in myself can make me confident in jumping off that ledge. No amount of self-soothing and other New Agey strategies of positive-thinking-produces-positive-outcomes bullshit would work here. But I look at what is scary, what is discomfiting, and I stare it down.

At Tough Mudder, I had a job to do, and I had to do it or face weeks of personal frustration and energy-sapping anger.

I steeled myself against the invisible but very palpable wall of fear and bumped against it a few times before the chanting and counting down of the folks below, who forced me to confront that wall and burst through it.

I jumped, free-falling and splashing into the murky water below. I don't remember the freefall, or what it felt like. I don't even remember if I had my eyes closed or not. I recall the initial sensation of jumping and the acute fear of not being in control, of being uncomfortable.

I don't have a fear of heights. In fact, I love them. Mountaintops and cliff edges enchant me. I'm drawn to high, shaky bridges over gorges with steep drops. Even skydiving and hang gliding fascinate me. Standing on ledges and looking down beneath me doesn't inspire a deep fear within me. Precisely the loss of control causes a fear so deep. I'm not a control freak, nor am I one of those people who enjoy being in the limelight for the simple act of being in it.

I jumped. And they cheered. I swam to the edge and climbed out of the muddy water.

This is what I love: the instant camaraderie and the deep, almost immediate friendships formed by the common goal of surpassing our own low expectations, jumping into uncertainty, and doing what we thought was impossible. This has been my journey.

But a journey denotes some kind of movement, travel—it means some type of motility—some movement along a spectrum, if you will. Inertia never sat well with me. I always preferred some part of my body to be moving. If it wasn't my legs running and jumping outside, doing fence races with my cousins, it was moving my eyes, devouring books. Always moving, with sense, with purpose, progressing along the spectrum of human possibility.

25

FLAWLESS

Wow! Oh shit! You have eyebrows," my sister, Allie, exclaimed as she inspected my made-up face. "I didn't even recognize you. Oh shit, lemme find out, though!"

I had met Allie and my mom for dinner at Columbus Circle on a warm spring night in April of 2016.

"Mirna, they *did* your face. They, like, fucking created a new person," she continued in disbelief. "Oh shit! Wow! I can't even believe you have *brows*, girl. *Brows*. When was the last time you had brows?"

"Um, never."

"Yeah, I know." Allie laughed. "But you look good, sis. I'm proud of you. Wow!"

"Thanks. I've never had my makeup done, like, professionally. This is weird. I feel crazy. I feel like a fat doll. Like, not in a bad way. But this is different."

I had flown from Georgia to participate in a photo shoot featuring plus-sized models such as Hayley Hasselhoff and Alessandra Garcia-Lorido. It was the brainchild of the folks at Evans, a British fashion company catering to plus-sized women.

I pushed the "Up" button for the elevator and waited for what seemed like an eternity for the industrial-sized metal-box elevator to whisk me upstairs. The studio was airy and brightly lit, but the incandescent track lighting only highlighted and made warmer the somewhat harsh but glimmering light reflecting off the Hudson River.

What is this? I asked myself. *How did this happen? How the heck am I about to do this?*

I stepped off the elevator, looked around, and a tall, skinny, well-dressed, and coiffed British man rushed over and embraced me. He was wearing tight and faded jeans, a scarf, and pointy black shoes to go with his wavy, gelled blond hair.

"O.M.G," he said. "Look who just came off the lift! She's here! I'm Tom, and I can't tell you how excited we are that you're here! Can I get you some coffee? A muffin? Anything? Let me take you over to where you'll be in hair and makeup. Oh my God, this is so exciting!"

How is this all happening right here right now? How am I standing (awkwardly and just a tad overwhelmed) in this big New York studio waiting for hair and makeup? Is this for real? This was no glamour photo shoot at the local mall. This was the real deal, with a famous photographer who shoots famous people.

Danielle Levitt, the celebrity photographer, was running shit and her right-hand woman, Stephanie, was running around, ensuring that everyone was where they were supposed to be and no time or space was wasted, that everyone looked the way Danielle envisioned them in the final product. She arranged the Uber rides, the schedules, the props, the caterers . . . *Oh, the caterers! I could do this for a living,* I said to myself. *Have wholesome but sumptuously fancy catered food delivered to me while I work at just being me in a beautiful space in the Village?* I'll take it. Warm quinoa with lemon and parsley, strip steak, Mediterranean chicken in some delectable sauce. Olive-oil cake? *What? I'll take that too.*

Isabel, the organizational superstar on the Evans side of the shoot, directed me to a low chair to sit and wait for a few minutes before it was my turn for hair and makeup. I had no idea the extent to which I was about to be transformed into not another person but an extremely different, more poignant version of myself. She began cleaning my face, stripping it of any dirt and oil that had accumulated on my ride from the chic hotel in tourist-ridden Times Square.

The lead makeup artist looked at my face, turning my chin ever so slightly with her forefinger. "Flawless," she exclaimed in a very London-like accent. "Flawless! But we need to do something about these brows. Do you mind if we fix up the brows a bit?"

"Pluck all of this away, and then shape up here," she directed one of the assistants who stood next to me. "Clean this up a bit too? Okay, just flawless," she said as she tipped my head up again to admire my blemish-free dark-chocolate skin.

My eyes began to water as Natalia, the assistant makeup artist assigned to transform my virgin face into a work of art worthy of high fashion, plucked away, for such was the price of fashion-industry-approved beauty. I don't think I could ever become accustomed to pulling the hairs out of my face, but maybe that comes with age? Perhaps, but I'm not yet ready for that.

Natalia was of Portuguese origin, small and petite, but fast, strong, and extraordinarily talented. She took advantage of all her makeup tools: the powders, compressed or creamy; the creams, thick or thin; the lotions, liquids, brushes, foam triangles, cotton balls, Q-tips, sprays and mists, oils, towels, lipsticks, glosses, shimmery and clear creamy substances. The color palette ranged from a very light peach, almost white, to dark brown, to shades even darker than my own skin, to almost black. There were oranges and pinks and purples, blues, grays, and metallics. There was a range of what I like to think of as instruments of torture: eyelash curlers, pluckers, tweezers, scissors, little and big brushes that I just *knew* would give me an allergic reaction.

Danielle, a native of Los Angeles, was short and thin with blond, artsy hair in tight curls. The camera flash clicked a thousand times per second. *How did they pick me? Why did they pick me?* This was a world that most people only dream of being part of, this world of photographers milling about, assistants scurrying around and heeding orders, caterers veering in and out, feeding the vast amount of people required to take a photo of a couple of women dressed in fancy clothing.

What was I doing here, anyway, with real-life professional models? My feet were fucked up royally—ugly runner's feet that looked like runner's feet before I even started running in high school. Didn't they know this? Hadn't they seen my unibrow or my one bucktooth?

They patted and pulled, brushed, and wiped for about two hours until my face was ready. The lead artist came over and started issuing orders.

"Can you put a little more color here? And more orange on the cheeks?" She peered at me again. "Also, less matte and glisten on the lips. Wait, maybe no more matte, and just a little gloss. More definition in the brows; she has such lovely brows and flawless skin. Just *flawless*."

Natalia and Aya, another assistant, worked tirelessly on my face, creating a version of me that I didn't know existed. I caught glimpses of my reflection in the mirror (when my eyes weren't watering from the eyelash curler). I didn't recognize myself.

Kendall, the hairdresser, worked on the tousled and damaged mess that was my hair.

"All these split ends? *Gurrrrllll*," he said, frowning, shaking his braided head, and clicking his tongue. "No excuse. No excuse for this. You could at least get a trim once a month. And what is all this product? I'll take care of it today, but you are under strict orders to wash your hair three times tonight. You'll condition it, and then let it air-dry. Absolutely no product whatsoever, because I just *can't* with that, okay? And then I'll do what I can. Now you know for next time."

Wow! I looked runnerly, but I also felt a different kind of beautiful—strong, powerful, appreciated, noticed, and loved. I was in a New York City studio being photographed because I represented something a *fashion* company saw as inspirational to them and possibly to other women. I kept looking around in wonderment.

All of us had individual time with Danielle, and she chatted with each girl to help even the professionals warm up.

"So you're the runner?"

"Yep!"

"Wow, I read about you. You do, like, marathons and ultramarathons. What possesses you to do such crazy stuff? I can barely do three miles." She had clearly done her homework and made sure to tell the right story with her photos and videos, poses, and facial expressions. She was funny and made me laugh.

"Show a little bit of attitude," she directed. "Feel like the badass you are."

This only made me laugh more. "Um, okay, I'm a badass." I felt less awkward and unnatural, and after a while I loosened up.

"Move forward and backward. Then move side to side. Give me a little hip."

"Like this?" I asked.

"Yeah, give me a little more and move your arms too. You're a little stiff right now, girl."

"I have no idea what I'm doing!" I moved to the left, then to the right.

"Girl, you look great! Stephanie, look at these!"

"Now look up at the light. Look over there a little. Hug yourself."

I tried to follow her directions as they came, but she was quick. The only breaks I had were when the lead hairstylist tousled my hair a little more, or when Natalia or Aya rushed up to redo my lipstick.

"Okay, now profile, your left shoulder to me. Look at me and smile. Now smile with your eyes. A little more hip. *Yesssss!* That's it!"

Click, click, click.

The whole process took two full days: more makeup, more hairstyling, and more clothing, shoes, and accessories. More flashing, more delicious catered goodies, and more people rushing about, shushing us, praising us, and telling us that we, plus-sized women, were gorgeous and worthy.

Even for someone like me, who has a strong sense of self and a streak of confidence that can seem a little much for some, having folks in the beauty and fashion industry refer to me as *flawless* hit a good nerve, pushing me further along that continuum of self-love and acceptance.

26

A BEAUTIFUL WORK IN PROGRESS

My fourteen-year-old son, Rashid, is the kind of child-cum-teenager-but-still-a-child that puts sprigs of lemon thyme in his homemade lemonade complete with lemon slices and pulp ("You *have* to have the pulp, Mom!"); asks for tapenade when pretzel chips are served; makes his mom a fried egg, Gruyère, applewood-smoked bacon, and spinach stack with gluten-free toast for Mother's Day; and insists that Shirazes are better than Malbecs—"well, because they are, Mom."

They just are . . . He is the kind of kid who still asks for cuddle time at the most busy and inopportune moments, falls asleep to the Disney channel (I *can't* explain this one), tries to hide it when he is feeling emotional pain, and knocks me over with his overbearing yet bony and muscular "I am taller than you, Mom" bear hugs—and I'm a pretty solid, strong woman.

He is *also* the kind of recently turned teenager who is able to live in smelly squalor with plastic wrappings from I don't know what, empty and sticky bottles, plates with all kinds of grossness soldered to them by darkness and age, clothes he couldn't and wouldn't find after stuffing them in between his bed and the wall, and dirty socks—all under his bed. He will *try* to wear the same underwear he had on before his long bath—"But I only had them on for a few hours, Mom"—tries to ignore me when he's eating meals with his friends in our school's dining hall (but I make sure to run over and give him very loud kisses so that he remains on the edge of slight mortification). He also needs reminding to actually *do* his homework, to shower after sports, and to clean up after himself every single time. He's a complex kid. He's an absolutely normal, albeit quirky, human being, like most of us are.

Rashid is growing and changing, learning something new every day and experimenting with his newfound knowledge and experiences. Sometimes he reverts to his childlike ways (whining, pouting, and clamoring loudly for attention), and other times he exhibits a seriously sardonic adult side that makes me shiver. His brain is experiencing exponential growth, as is his entire body, morphing him into an almost-six-foot-tall, lanky human being.

This newly minted teenager is allowed to experiment and change, sometimes under the critical eyes of society. At school and adolescent-friendly places, he's encouraged to grow and make mistakes repeatedly, supported when he falls, and given a hand when he needs help to try something again, to try something new.

Sometimes I wish I were still that awkward, pudgy, extremely shy thirteen-year-old standing at the start line of the mile at the boarding school that helped change the trajectory of my life. The world was my oyster and I felt it. I knew implicitly that I was free to explore, change, experiment, and morph into the human being that I was supposed to be, whatever that was. I'm still trying to figure out what and who I want to be when I grow up.

Why are complexity and flexibility so problematic for adults? As a forty-plus-year-old, I'd like to think that I'm always standing at the precipice of change and progress, that I'm constantly on a ledge facing a wall of fear—a wall that, if I don't break it intentionally, will hinder my evolution and stop my personal growth. If I don't make peace with the thunderstorm that seeks to put me in my place, I'll be stuck cowering under a rock, rotting and dying.

I'd like to think that most of us are moving toward something, somewhere, or at least if we aren't, we're open to the idea that if we're stuck, maybe we should try something new, something else. What we are now is not what we were. Where we are now is not where we will be, unless we *want* to continue existing in the same reality over and over again.

What we are now can be vastly different from what we want or need to be. But each individual journey is a process—a unique way of being in the world, an exclusively human undertaking that is fraught with back stepping, stagnation, plateauing, and, perhaps most importantly, moving forward on the continuum toward greatness.

We're always heading somewhere, and I want to believe that most people want to be going in the direction that is best for them. Sure, not all people believe that they can progress into the being that they want or need to be, but my hope is that most of us are aiming and working to be our best selves most of the time.

The reason I began this journey, or more accurately, continued on it after a rather long hiatus, was threefold:

I had a health wake-up call that brought attention to the fact that I was stymied physically and mentally, and I was on my way to an early death.

I began to progress again, as I reacquainted myself with the forward movement that is running.

In addition, my health returned, and my smile became genuine again.

———

I started writing my blog *Fat Girl Running* not because I wanted or needed notoriety and validation, but because I needed an outlet to write about what I was experiencing at the time. I didn't think I was unique in that I was a fat girl who ran, but I thought I could get some leverage out of the name of the blog and its content, which would be about this one fat girl's journey in running. Early on, I made it a point to let my readers know that it wouldn't be a weight-loss blog, although I would mention it from time to time. I didn't want it to become some sob story about how I was so fat that I couldn't move like a human was supposed to. I also didn't want people to pity me because I was fat . . . there was no need. I was plenty confident and pretty self-assured. And I had already lost a significant amount of weight. I wanted to share my progress and my movement along the continuum of health and wellness while I continued to live, breathe, and exist happily in the body that I inhabit.

I wanted to share these experiences I was having while running. Although I had never taken to meditation, I was well aware of its benefits. Running was my meditation. It allowed me to empty my mind and focus on my own footfalls, my breathing. I would briefly look ahead to keep on track, but then I would get back into my own head and be in the moment. In my crazy world of working at boarding school I was finding the need to get off campus and engage in routine self-care. Working in a place that operates on a twenty-four-hour schedule can make self-care difficult, especially as a woman with a family. I found myself again on this journey, welcoming a new and urgent sense of health and wellness of mind, body, and spirit.

Most of the time, when I'm not wallowing in the depths of self-pity or self-loathing, I'm *striving* to be the best person I can be. Whether that means attending workshops and conferences to improve my teaching, reflecting on a parenting decision I've made, trying hard to reverse the health trajectory of my family, or confronting issues in my marriage, I'm constantly looking to be and do better. I fail many times, but this frequent failure means there's always vast room for modification and improvement, which is what drives me to keep doing what I do.

In no way do I believe that simply becoming thin and aspiring to look like what mainstream media messages suggest I should look like will make me happier. Will losing weight help lessen the likelihood that I'll suffer from the chronic illnesses that continue to plague my family? Maybe. Will it lessen the stress I am placing on my joints? Absolutely.

I become emotionally drained by living in a body whose shape is assumed to be the product of indolence, letting myself go (whatever that means), lack of self-control, intellectual and moral inferiority, and surrendering to the primordial urgencies of hunger. I am complex. I am more than what my body suggests to others visually.

According to the fat-person stereotype, I'm supposed to sit on my big fat ass at a desk all day (if I work at all), with a forty-ounce plastic cup of soda by my side. I'm supposed to inhale one, maybe two fourteen-inch supreme pizzas while in front of the television, trapped on a couch. I'm supposed to waddle and be unwieldy, tripping over my own fat feet.

I'm supposed to be constantly out of breath, reaching for the asthma inhaler that only prolongs my suffering. I'm supposed to be beholden to all sorts of body fluid–regulating medications: one for high blood pressure, one for pancreatic malfunction, one for excess fluid in my legs, one for the proper release or suppression of hormones, one for kidney issues, and another for constricted arteries.

I'm definitely *not* supposed to be out in public, anywhere really, unless I'm visiting a bariatric surgery center. I'm *not* supposed to be in any kind of restaurant, even the hip and esoteric salad bars with names like Green Leaf and Health Box Minimalist Tasteless Bullshit, because I'm not supposed to be eating at *all*.

I'm not supposed to be hiking, but I do. I'm not supposed to be at the gym, but I go. I shouldn't be, but I do. And God forbid I actually undress and show my naked fat body in the gym locker room. I may be photographed. I may become a viral social-media post, at the expense of myself. And I'm definitely not supposed to be running outside in front of people enjoying myself *without* an obsession about losing the weight I carry on *my* body. I'm not supposed to be on this mountain or that hill, hanging by a rope, outfitted in a climbing harness. I'm too big, I'm too fat, I'm too . . .

I'm not supposed to be in a bathing suit or bikini near *any* body of water. I should be in a tent dress, where no part of my apparently unsightly body can be seen. I'm not supposed to be a sponsored athlete who gets to do really cool things in the name of sport in my fat body. And honestly, I have no *business* having an ambassadorship with a major outdoor company because there are so many "fit" people who work out and "Why are you getting all this attention? You're just doing it for the attention!" I'm not supposed to be showing my *photos* on social media, because how dare I create my own fitness narrative that isn't centered on weight loss? How dare I *not* focus on changing parts of my body that are deemed aesthetically displeasing?

I'm not supposed to be proud of my body and all that it can do. How obnoxious of me to appear as though I matter? I'm fat, after all; that is, lazy, slovenly, and not worthy of being loved, liked, or admired. Bottom line is, I simply should cease to exist.

But that's all wrong. I have a body that is amazing and strong. It's flexible and agile. It can carry me across one hundred kilometers and up and down mountains. It has birthed a baby and survived fractures, breaks, and multiple bouts of pneumonia.

It can do yoga and Tough Mudders. It was deemed worthy enough to be featured in *Runner's World*, the *Wall Street Journal*, and *NBC Nightly News*. It was seen as beautiful and athletic when I was invited to do a photo shoot with professional plus-size models for Evans clothing. It was accepted as athletic and donned with the appropriately sporty high-end clothing of Merrell, Swiftwick, and Skirt Sports.

This body isn't meant to stagnate or cease moving. When we stop moving in mind, body, and spirit, we stop learning. When we stop learning, we stop living. Therefore, when we stop moving, we stop living. We stop evolving toward being the humans we are destined to be.

This body is fierce, beautiful, and unapologetic. It's meant to move through the world as it wishes: lifting, walking, and running, rolls and all. Love handles, bouncy boobs, curves, tummy, butt, back fat, and all. I honor her by continuing to move along the spectrum of health and wellness, and in turn she honors me by living vibrantly.

> *Fat girl running, swimming,*
> *moving, learning, pausing, progressing,*
> *jiggling, rubbing, chafing, shaking,*
> *sinking, rising, living,*
> *being.*

APPENDIX

THE FATASS BADASS ATHLETE

In September of 2016, I was invited to speak at the Fat Activism Conference, created by Ragen Chastain and other prominent body-positive activists. I relished the opportunity to speak truth to power to other women who might question their right to be athletes. As Bill Bowerman, one of the cofounders of Nike, said, "If you have a body, you're an athlete." This was my speech in full.

BECOMING, BEING, AND CELEBRATING THE ATHLETE YOU'VE ALWAYS BEEN IN THE BODY YOU HAVE

Before I begin, I'll tell you a little bit about myself.

Again, my name is Mirna Valerio. I'm originally from Brooklyn, New York, but currently live in the Appalachian Mountains in northeast Georgia. I am the director of equity and inclusion, a Spanish teacher, and cross-country coach at the Rabun Gap Nacoochee School, a boarding school. In my "free time" I am a marathoner, ultramarathoner, nascent obstacle-course racer, blogger at *Fat Girl Running* and *Women's Running Magazine*. I'm also writing a running memoir called *A Beautiful Work in Progress*, due for publication in October of 2017.

I have a spouse—he is from Burkina Faso in West Africa—and a very handsome and snarky thirteen-year-old whose only concerns right now are basketball and when's the next time he can eat Grandma's food. Between playing basketball, soccer, and tennis, and swimming, they're both pretty phenomenal athletes.

My life is radically different now than it was just under two years ago.

In January of 2015, I was contacted by Rachel Bachman, a fitness and health writer at the *Wall Street Journal* who had been reading my blog *Fat Girl Running* and was wondering if she could interview me about a piece she was doing entitled "Weight Loss or Not, Exercise Has Benefits." That piece was published a week later, and it rocked my world. Traffic to my blog increased, and then John Brant, from *Runner's World*, e-mailed me and asked if I would be amenable to them doing a feature on me.

On me? Wait, on me? A fat girl? In Runner's World? *Hells yeah!*

That piece was published in the August 2015 issue of *Runner's World*, and my life was turned upside down, in a very, very good way.

NBC Nightly News picked up the story and then my world blew up, also in a very, *very* good way.

Now, I would like to share some of the goodness I have reaped from living a pretty public life as a fat athlete. And I have to tell you, it has been great to be part of a movement that I *didn't even know existed* until last year.

I seriously was not aware that there was such a thing as the Health at Every Size movement, or a fat-activism movement, or even a formal Body Positive Movement. But now more than ever, there is an urgent need to embrace ourselves, who we are right now, *how* we are right now, and kick ass while we're doing it, in the pursuit of pure, unbridled athleticism.

So this is how I'm here today speaking to you about how you, too, can embrace the athleticism you've always had within you but maybe didn't know how to access. Or maybe you've been discouraged because of the culture of fat-hate we've all been subjected to, whether we're fat or not. Or maybe you're just looking for a way to practice or grow your self-acceptance and body-love. Unlocking the athlete in you is one way to achieve this!

In this workshop, you'll learn how to lead the authentically athletic and athletically authentic life you've always wanted to lead but didn't know how. I'll take you through my own process of becoming an athlete in *this. Body. Right. Here.* Then I'll walk you through a few steps so that you're able to come up with a plan to *own* and *celebrate* your own unabashed and fabulous athleticism. We'll talk gear, training, and mindset so you'll be able to lace up and go with confidence. Finally, we'll share wisdom learned through moving the bodies we have right now.

I believe that everyone who is able should move his or her body in an athletic way. For the health benefits and the simple badassery that comes along with moving your body intentionally.

Here are a few benefits of physical activity, according to the CDC:

- Reducing risk of some cancers and diseases (such as colon and breast cancer, cardiovascular disease, and type 2 diabetes)
- Strengthening your bones and muscles
- Improving your mental health and mood
- Improving your ability to perform daily activities (functional strength and flexibility)
- Increasing your chances of living longer

We all know these things. *Blah, blah, blah.*

But what about embracing the lifestyle of an athlete? Until this revolution in body image began, no one talked to us fat people about becoming athletes in the bodies that we have. It was always, "Maybe you can be an athlete after you lose X amount of pounds or maybe after you become what many consider aesthetically acceptable in body, then you can be an athlete."

This is not true. Of course we know that intellectually, but some of us are still trepidatious about taking those first steps to being an athlete.

So . . . What about taking that huge step *now*, a step that may seem out of reach for some, by calling ourselves the athletes that we are now, or can be? How about it?

Believing is being. Being is believing.

Here are the benefits of being an *athlete*, and taking your physical fitness to the next level. These are the observations that I've noticed about myself personally and have discovered in my research as well:

- When you start seeing yourself as an athlete, negative self-talk diminishes, allowing you to see individual workouts/regimens as part of a larger goal for lifelong fitness and health!
- Training as an athlete helps you become agile and flexible, not only physically, but mentally too.
- You begin to have a mutually respectful relationship with your body. You honor it by working it, by strengthening it and making it more flexible. And in turn, your body honors you by carrying you with strength and flexibility throughout your life.
- You begin to know your body intimately. You begin to feel where mental and emotional distress is manifesting in your body. And then, hopefully, you are more prepared to deal with those issues that hamper your happiness.
- You become more adventurous. When your body is primed, strong, and ready for new things, your mind will follow.
- Calling yourself an athlete makes you accountable to yourself.

Kristen Dieffenbach, a sports psychologist and associate professor of athletic coaching education at West Virginia University, says,

"Calling yourself an 'athlete' can play an important role in how you see yourself and how you ultimately perform."

Dieffenbach continues, "There's an intrinsic value you get in terms of a sense of pride and feeling good about your commitment. That's the core of being an athlete, whether it's for a medal or just to say, 'Yep, I did that.'"

Finally, although his website and book are geared toward a specific audience, one that is primarily male and focused on a traditionally "athletic" look, I love the following reasons Eric Bach, fitness professional and author, gives to train like an athlete (which, interestingly enough, downplay the whole idea of a certain body aesthetic).

From Bachperformance.com, those reasons are:

1. Improved athletic performance
2. Improved versatility
3. Improved conditioning
4. Improved work capacity—as in the ability to lift heavier things both at the gym and at home—and this decreases those nagging little injuries that inhibit our functional movement, especially as we age (like throwing out your back, for example)
5. Fewer imbalance injuries: for the same reasons above. Any intense work of all sets of muscles increases our strength and flexibility in all planes. So thrown-out back, dead-butt syndrome, and frozen shoulder be damned!

So why is this presentation even necessary? Why would anyone want to listen to *me* talk about becoming an athlete? We're constantly bombarded with messages that fat people cannot be athletes, and sometimes we as fat people even believe that bullshit.

Last year I was the keynote speaker at a wonderful event in Portland, Oregon, sponsored by Heart to Start, an organization that encourages everyone in every body to walk, run, and strength-train for the betterment of their physical and mental lives. Here's a bit of what I said back then:

- Our bodies are designed to move and to be outside. We are built to be physically active. All of us. And to that end, we must love, honor, accept, and respect our bodies as they are, while constantly striving for improvement.
- We can only be our authentic selves; it is too physically and emotionally exhausting to try to be something that we are not. When we are not being authentic, our whole selves lose out on life.
- Our physical health and well-being are intrinsically and intimately related to our mental, emotional, and spiritual wealth and health.
- Physical fitness is not the exclusive purview of people who appear to be physically fit. Get outside, show up for yourself, and show your body to the world.
- Keep a journal or a training log so that you can look back at your progress and say to yourself, "I did that," or conversely, look at yourself critically and say, "I need to do better."
- Know that you will have low points on your journey. You might hallucinate. You might literally run into a cactus. You might suffer from an injury. Life will happen. In fact, you will have really low points in which you will ask yourself, "Why am I doing this?" Or you'll say to yourself, "I'm not seeing any *results*." You'll wonder why you even bother. You might even doubt your sanity. You will come upon both major and minor obstacles and hurdles on your course. But as I have learned countless times from being on the pavement or on the trail for hours and hours at a time, you have no choice but to overcome the hurdles or modify your course. But you must keep moving forward. There is no turning back on your health, on

yourself. Let's continue giving ourselves and others the gift of health and wellness, and ultimately—and, I think, most importantly—it is my belief that everyone who is able should pursue exercise in an athletic way, because of all that I've mentioned up to now, and also because that's what human bodies are designed for. Movement. Pure and simple.

It's time to break this habit, to break the mold and unleash that fierce, unstoppable, strong athlete that you've always been.

So let's start.

This talk is actually an extended version of a very popular post from my blog *Fat Girl Running*, "How to Be a Fatrunner in Ten Simple Steps."

So now, in the name of general athleticism and badassery, here is *how* to become a *Fatass Badass Athlete* in ten simple steps:

1. **Embrace the title of ATHLETE.** A lot of times, nomenclature or semantics make decisions for us. It's time to take the name of athlete and *do* something with it. Use it as a weapon, a sign you proudly wear across your forehead and fatass to let people know who you are and what awesomeness you are about to achieve, what amazingness you are or will be able to accomplish. LIVE IT. Be proud. Be active. EMBRACE the name, embrace your body, and LOVE it.

2. **Decide to BE an athlete.** Whether it's running, walking, sprinting, climbing, doing CrossFit, becoming an OCR [obstacle course race] fanatic, morphing yourself into a yogi, doing track-and-field events, swimming, cycling, or training for your first or hundredth triathlon—working hard at these things and being committed and disciplined in your training automatically qualify you as an athlete. However, YOU and only YOU can make the decision to be one. It's really not up to anyone but YOU.

3. **Have a practice of visual and visceral self-love**. Look in the mirror and smile, even if it doesn't feel genuine. Sometimes we have to fake it until we make it. Literally embrace yourself, hug your body, and then thank your body for how it has supported you thus far. Make a promise to your body that you will honor and nourish it, as it has honored and nourished you.

4. **State and chant your mantra**. Have a favorite mantra? Now is your opportunity to repeat it several times. What is it? If you don't already have one, here are a few to use until you do:

- I like this one from Dr. Christiane Northrup, the renowned women's health expert, but no doubt this mantra is for people of all gender identities: "I love myself unconditionally right now." Let's practice: I love myself unconditionally right now. I love myself unconditionally right now. I love myself unconditionally right now.
- Another favorite mantra came to me while I was running a tough 35M race in the northern Georgia mountains. I was wet, tired, extremely hungry, and DONE. But then when the moment came that I questioned why I was doing this to myself, voluntarily I might add, I stopped and gained some perspective. I realized that even though I was at a low point, and that I still had about sixteen more grueling and mountainous miles to go, I was able to move freely, in a beautiful forest, propelling my own body forward. There are people who don't get to spend inordinate amounts of time moving their bodies in the way they want or need to. There are also people who are so disenchanted with their lives that they are stuck physically and emotionally. At that point in my life, I was grateful to not be experiencing any of those things. I was and am grateful to be living the dream. So I said to myself (and I say to myself

quite often), I AM LIVING THE DREAM. I am living the dream. I. Am. Living. The. Dream. LIVE YOUR DREAM.

- Yet another mantra I frequently use is: **GET IT DONE. JUST GET IT DONE.** This is me being a teacher and coach to myself. Do the work. Get it done. Because there really is no other option when you have big goals and plans like crossing the finish line at a big race, or lifting three hundred pounds or simply enjoying pure athleticism. There have certainly been times when I have not finished doing all the work for various reasons: I knew that my race was over, the race director said that my race was over, or if I pressed on, there would be long-lasting physical consequences, like not being able to drive myself home or function the next day. Otherwise, I get it done.

6. This will be the longest one so far: **Put on your workout clothes!** Many of us larger folks have some issues finding workout clothing that is (1) comfortable and (2) does not make us feel (or look) like a link of brats that is about to explode, or a bear in a big, ugly tent. This is a major conundrum that *must* be dealt with or it might cause us to have an excuse to not get out there and be badass as we should be doing every day. I have had constant issues with finding comfortable, nonpinching or cinching outfits that make me feel and look good. When you can wear something that feels awesome on you, you kind of exude awesomeness. Although compared to, say, ten years ago, the offerings have increased a hundredfold, there are still not enough retailers and designers who keep us curvy folks in mind when creating beautiful, functional, and sport-specific lines of clothing. I would *love* to be able to pop into "name a store" and magically fit into some oh-so-beautiful-sleek-and-form-fitting compression tights and jackets, but apparently that is not going to happen anytime soon, or ever. Some companies have made a

concerted effort to provide affordable and flattering sports clothing for us: Old Navy, Champion, and some big-name brands like Adidas and Nike are the first that come to mind—but I have found that the durability of those products is not on par with clothing for smaller folks. Do they expect us not to jump up and down, or move? Do they know that things jiggle and cause pants and shirts to bunch up, fall down, get stuck under tummies, and/or cause wedgies? DON'T THEY KNOW? I made the decision a while back to embrace my curves, wear form-fitting workout clothing that actually fits, and to look at myself in the mirror every single day and think at least one positive thought. This has made me appreciate my body in clothes. But it takes the right clothes—you know, pieces that don't look like you're in a parachute, or hot-air balloon . . . or in jail—to achieve this.

- So do you only have sweats or jeans? Yoga pants or cargo pants? Have a favorite T-shirt that makes you feel and act fabulous? WHATEVER, they're workout clothes so put them on.
- On the other hand, having some excellent, high-quality workout clothing will make a huge difference in the way that you feel before, during, and after your workout. The great thing about being fat AND being an athlete these days is that there is actually athletic clothing designed with us in mind. Granted, we are still at the beginning of the fashion and athletic apparel industries being totally inclusive size-wise, but we are getting somewhere.
- As I said, there are a host of companies that cater to us and I'll include a whole list of those in the supplementary materials. Also, if you head over to my blog, you'll see posts dedicated specifically to workout apparel and shoe reviews for us.
- So make a time investment to research and try on different clothing, and then make a financial investment for good

quality gear that will allow you to comfortably (and fashion-ably, if that's your thing) do your workout.

- If you don't have workout clothing yet, NO FEAR! Work out in whatever you have, without embarrassment, fear, or a second thought! It can be prohibitively expensive to get quality gear, so until then and until you are financially able, do with what you've got!

- I am fortunate to have had my world change in the last two years. If you're like me, you've always had issues finding clothing that fits, is functional and flattering in color, style, and cut. On a personal note, I no longer have to deal with this issue. I am a sponsored athlete. No, really! This fat girl, RIGHT HERE, is a sponsored athlete. In addition to repping Swiftwick socks, I have two high-profile relationships with Merrell and Skirt Sports. Never in my dreams did I think I would be able to attend sports events, decked out in functional clothing that actually fit me, representing various athletic apparel companies, IN MY BIG-ASS BODY, doing things that many people think I cannot do.

7. **Look in the mirror AGAIN**, and this time admire yourself for being a Badass Fatass Athlete. Repeat your mantra again several times until you start believing it or until you start feeling crazy. Either totally works. Say to yourself: I AM AN ATHLETE. I AM A FATASS BADASS ATHLETE. I am an athlete. I. AM. AN. ATHLETE.

8. **Work out. GO HARD OR GO HOME**. Most of the time—okay, sometimes you'll be exhausted. That's okay. That said, athletes are defined by their dedication and skill in whatever sport they're engaged in. Make sure you are committed. Make sure training becomes not only part of your everyday life (whether it's actual training or rest and recovery) but part of the fabric of your life. When I say, go hard or go home, I'm not talking about training to

the point of injury. Obviously, we want to avoid injury at all costs, because let me tell you, being injured sucks. It sucks the life out of all that you've done to achieve where you are in your training, and it is also a huge mental mountain looming ahead in the distance. Really, what I'm talking about is not only being completely and totally committed to athleticism but also committed to the idea of you yourself achieving athletic greatness. It is about the preparation and journey as well as the product, be it a marathon, getting significantly stronger, logging a truly epic bike ride, kayaking down a really long, winding river with rapids, nailing a difficult dance routine, competing in that two-mile open-water swim, teaching a fitness class, or whatever! It takes a serious belief in yourself and a commitment to excellence even through the pretty extreme lows that you will undoubtedly have.

9. **Take selfies and pics to record these momentous occasions, to share with your friends and family.** So that you can see the awesomeness of who you are and what you do often. Get used to looking at yourself and admiring what's there and what your body can do. That energy will radiate from you to other folks and come back to you manifold! I once wrote the following on my blog in a post entitled "Selfie-Affirmation": I selfie every day that I run or do something that challenges my big, strong body. Sometimes I am alone, and other times I am with a group of people, both new friends and old. Sometimes I am in the midst of a particularly challenging exploit, and I will take a photo to remind myself that what I am doing is supposed to be hard, and I am actually *doing* it. I want my circles of family and friends to know what I've been up to, and how I look, even when the photo is not at all flattering. I want them to know that if there is something that inspires and motivates them, they should do it and snap photos of themselves doing that difficult thing too.

10. **Many people are asthmatic or have some underlying health concerns, like autoimmune disease, diabetes, and other illnesses.** Please check with a doctor you trust to guide you through the initial stages of your burgeoning athleticism. That said, be wary of anyone who dismisses your goals and dreams and feeds you canned and erroneous statements like "running will ruin your joints," or "you should lose weight before you start to work out," or "just go on a diet." Because seriously, did you listen to me at all? Please let all the folks in your medical team know what you're doing so that everyone's on the same page and on board. There are many successful fat athletes who are doing the same thing and have lots of support behind them. For example, I have a great nurse practitioner and doctor team that know I run marathons and work out a lot. They are 100 percent on board, and when I come in, the doctor's visit is framed in that way. I often hear the NP talking outside of the examination room door, prepping various nursing students: "Our next patient is an ultramarathoner and she's having some hip soreness," or "She has a bad sinus infection that she needs to get rid of before her 100K." This way, things are clear, and I am treated seriously as an athlete with medical needs.

11. **Do the thing.** Do yoga. Run your 5K or marathon. CrossFit to your heart's desire. Throw the discus. Swim your mile. Cycle your century. Jump over and own those obstacles. And do it again. But NOW, as a Badass Fatass Athlete.

And here is my final message to you:

Many of us are dealing with the repercussions of a fat-shaming, body-hating society. Just because we're working out, running, lifting weights, cycling, swimming, or leading a Zumba class, it does *not* mean that we have a problem with our body image. When people allude to that in their thinly veiled criticism masquerading as compliments ("Good for you!" "Wow!" "That's impressive!"), it simply means that they have a problem with their body image. They could get some help. And you should continue in pursuit of athleticism no matter what people say. In the end, we love ourselves and our bodies. Maybe not all of us are fully aware of this, but we do. If we didn't love our bodies, we wouldn't have this commitment to ourselves. We wouldn't be doing this thing.

SUPPLEMENTARY MATERIALS

Finally, get to know the following Fatass Badass Athletes! There are many of us, but here are just a few to read about and gain a little bit of motivation from:

- Jessamyn Stanley: the amazing, award-winning yogi
- Laura Backus: triathlete and blogger at *A Fat Girl's Ironman Journey*
- Roz Mays: owner of Dangerous Curves, Plus Size Pole Competition
- Jill Angie: runner, triathlete, and author of *Running with Curves*
- Louise Green: triathlete and plus-size athletic trainer
- Amanda Bingson: Olympic-level track-and-field athlete
- Krista Henderson: triathlete and owner of Born to Reign Athletics
- Leah Gilbert: triathlete featured in *Athena Multisport Magazine*
- Derek Mitchell: a 5K runner/walker traveling the country, motivating people of all sizes to run
- Cheryl Haworth: Olympic weight lifter

Websites of athletic apparel companies that cater to or include us and our badass athletic pursuits:

- katiekactive.com
- www.torrid.com
- www.lanebryant.com
- www.breezeactivewear.com
- www.eddiebauer.com
- www.dearkates.com
- www.skirtsports.com
- www.junonia.com
- enell.com
- www.oldnavy.com
- www.evansusa.com
- www.movingcomfort.com
- www.panache-lingerie.com
- www.nike.com
- lineagewear.com/collections
- glamorise.com
- Target.com
- Danskin.com

Some of these companies are still in the process of developing and refining their collections, making them more inclusive and more representative of people with bodies like us. If you find a company that is doing the right thing, please let me know, and I'll make sure to publicize the hell out of it!

Thank you so much for allowing me to be part of your fatass badass athletic journey.

If you have any questions, please feel free to reach me in any of the following ways:

My blog: fatgirlrunning-fatrunner.blogspot.com
My Facebook page: www.facebook.com/fattgirlrunning/
On Instagram and Twitter: @themirnavator
And my e-mail: themirnavator@gmail.com

I look forward to hearing from you! And good luck on your journey to becoming a Fatass Badass Athlete!

ACKNOWLEDGMENTS

This book would not have been possible without the love, help, and support from my family: Joann Taylor, Allen Taylor Sr., Natasha Taylor, Allen Taylor Jr., Ellington Bennett, and Cito Nikiema. The most special thanks go to my handsome and talented son, Rashid, who suffered through many a late night and early morning lulled to sleep by the clicking of my computer keyboard.

My profound and humble thanks go to:

Kashene, Shamar, Sherene, and Akila, whose generosity of home and spirit has carried me through and across many Marine Corps Marathons, and particularly the last one; the day before I ran this race I actually finished writing this book with all of you surrounding me.

Jorge Valerio Castro, for always supporting and championing me from wherever your peripatetic wanderings deposited you.

Lakeisha Perryman, for showing me that grace and hope are always available in unlimited quantities if you simply believe they exist.

Nikki Buccello, for being willing to explore all things health and fitness that first summer.

The Rabun Gap Nacoochee School, for allowing me space and time to live out my dreams on your beautiful campus.

My generous colleagues and friends who were my first readers: Gayle Gawlik, Rebecca Smith, Maureen McGee, Beth Loveland,

Alice Jump, and Amy Cox—thank you for offering your most honest, insightful, and incisive feedback on my earliest drafts.

Nancy Theeman, Susan Daily, and Linda Borgersen—you all believed in me from our earliest musical moments together—my most profound thanks to you for believing in me and telling me that I was smart and full of untapped potential.

Rachel Bachman, John Brant, Clare Duffy, and George Itzhak, for drastically changing the trajectory of my life with their collective curiosity and genius.

Margaux Nissen Gray, publicist extraordinaire, for seeing inspiration where I thought there was none.

Merrell, Tough Mudder, Swiftwick, and Skirt Sports, thank you for giving this fat girl a chance to prove that all bodies matter.

Porscha Burke and Tanya McKinnon for planting the seed of this book.

My literary agents, Jane Dystel and Miriam Goderich, who believed in me from the start. I owe you my most profound gratitude.

Erin Calligan Mooney. Thank you for choosing me.

Chad Sievers, for digging in, taking this manuscript apart with the detailed eye and approach of an FBI agent, and forcing me to produce the best writing I could.

Finally, to Grandma, Greg, Sherry, and Eric: your spirits continue to inspire me in everything I do.

ABOUT THE AUTHOR

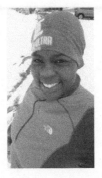

Mirna Valerio, a native of Brooklyn, New York, is a Spanish teacher, diversity practitioner, cross-country coach, ultrarunner, OCR enthusiast, and blogger. Valerio's blogs about all things running appear at *Fat Girl Running* and in *Women's Running Magazine*. Her story was featured in the *Wall Street Journal* and *Runner's World* and on *NBC Nightly News*. Valerio is a global ambassador for Merrell, an ambassador for Skirt Sports, and an athlete for Swiftwick. She is married to Cito Nikiema, and together they have a basketball-loving teenage son, Rashid. She loves being in nature and frequently runs trails in the northern Georgia mountains.